THE DEVELOPMENT OF COMMUNITY MENTAL HEALTH DIRECTORS:

A PHENOMENOLOGICAL STUDY

THE DEVELOPMENT OF COMMUNITY MENTAL HEALTH DIRECTORS:

A PHENOMENOLOGICAL STUDY

JERRY RAY STRAUSBAUGH

Gracednotes Ministries

Gracednotes Ministries

425 East Walnut Street

Ashland, Ohio 44805

The Development of Community Mental Health Directors:

A Phenomenological Study

Copyright by

Jerry Ray Strausbaugh

ISBN-13:978-1516807901

ISBN-10: 1516807901

A PHENOMENOLOGICAL STUDY OF THE DEVELOPMENTAL EXPERIENCE OF COMMUNITY MENTAL HEALTH DIRECTORS IN OHIO

BY

Jerry Ray Strausbaugh

ASHLAND UNIVERSITY, 2013

Constance Savage, Ph.D.

This dissertation is a study of the leadership development process of community mental health center (CMHC) executive directors in Ohio. CMHCs are tasked with providing services to individuals struggling with complex mental and emotional diagnoses. In Ohio these centers are nonprofit organizations that offer a multifaceted array of services paid for by a variety of third party funding sources. Many executive directors of Ohio CMHCs begin their careers as clinicians and must acquire the skills necessary to effectively lead their organization. In this study six Ohio CMHC executive directors who began their careers as clinicians were interviewed to discover the clinician-to-director developmental process. The data revealed two primary themes each with subthemes that describe the phenomenon experienced by the directors.

DEDICATION

This work is dedicated first to God who ordained it. I also dedicate it to my wife Jane who encouraged and supported me while also carrying the load at home, my daughters Melisa, Abby, and Krista who observed the whole process, and my parents Loren and Aldeth Strausbaugh who passed on their love, faith and values to me.

ACKNOWLEDGMENTS

I would like to sincerely thank the following people who had a major impact on my work and the ability to get this study accomplished:

To Dr. Constance Savage, my committee chair, who could see the completed product and guided me to the finish. Thank you for your support, wisdom, patience, and encouragement.

To Dr. James Olive for your knowledge of qualitative research and helping understand the best path for doing a phenomenological study.

To Dr. Alinde Moore for serving on my committee and for your adult development class which provided me with ideas and direction for my literature review and theoretical frame.

To Dr. Carla Edlefson, thank you for being such an encouragement during my entire time in the doctoral program.

To Susan Blake thank you for not only editing my work but also teaching me how to be a better writer.

To Jeff Pinkham, my library mentor, thank you for being so available and so helpful. Your practical understanding of the electronic-information-universe is remarkable.

To Teresa Lampl, thank you for sharing your knowledge of Ohio CMHCs and for helping me get started.

To Kim Calhoun, thank you for transcribing each interview.

To the Appleseed Community Mental Health Center Board of Directors, thank you for your encouragement and allowing me to have the time to complete this project.

To the staff and administration at Appleseed Community Mental Health Center, thank you for continuing to teach me so much about leadership.

To my father-in-law Terry Thomas, thank you for being such an encouragement and for all of the practical ways you help me.

To the six directors who participated in this study, thank you for opening up your lives and experiences to me. Thank you for genuinely telling your stories. May this work bless others who serve as directors of community mental health centers.

TABLE OF CONTENTS

There is no magic. There is only leadership, and ...
you give definition to what that looks like.
And for us it's an embracing of ideas and then a final voice ...
but the magic is, you know, opening the ears to the voices and to letting people
experience hearing their own voices.

a study participant

CHAPTER I

Introduction

For the last seven years I have been the executive director of a community mental health center (CMHC). I accepted this position after working as a family counselor for thirteen years. It quickly became apparent that the set of skills and perspectives that I needed to gain for this new position differed from what had made me a successful counselor and clinical supervisor. Not only did I have to learn about budgets, strategic planning, human resource management, and navigating politics but I also had to examine myself more than ever. To be the leader the agency needed, I had to gain a clear understanding of my strengths, weaknesses, fears, deficits, and gifts. I had to learn to apply what I knew about family systems to an organization. The experience that I had transitioning as a leader has given me a strong desire to better understand the experiences of other community mental health directors who move from being clinicians to being directors. By better understanding how the most effective leaders have developed through this experience and learning what helped them come through it successfully, I hope to be able to help others navigate their development more successfully.

My own professional training as a clinician fell short of preparing me for leading a mental health agency: That training, which was entirely clinical, did not include any instruction on how to manage and lead an organization. The phenomenon of clinicians developing in and adapting to the field of mental health leadership was identified as early as the 1970s, when Hirschowitz (1971) discussed the challenges of mental health directors. He described the difficulties that people with primarily clinical backgrounds faced on entering the leadership of community mental health as it was developing in the 1970s.

This work was a phenomenological study designed to explore the lived experience of CMHC executive directors who began their careers as clinicians. Van Manen (1990) has explained that to begin phenomenological study researchers must examine their own experience with the topic and explore their interest in it (pp. 30–31). My experience as a clinician-turned-director has given me an interest in exploring the phenomenon of leadership development experienced by mental health professionals becoming agency directors. At the time of writing this research project, I was in my eighth year as an agency director. Over the years the demands of the job have tested me psychologically, spiritually, intellectually, relationally, and professionally to the very core of my being. I am not the same person in any of those human domains as I was when I took the job in July 2005. I find that I have had to continually adapt, change, and grow, sometimes painfully, in order to meet the challenges of the role. By exploring the stories of other clinicians-turned-agency-directors I hope to provide a better understanding of the phenomenon so that new leaders can draw strength for the job by knowing how others successfully navigated these sometimes tempestuous waters.

Statement of the Problem

The field of American mental health administration began in 1773 with the opening of the country's first psychiatric hospital. James Gault was named as the "keeper" of the Virginia Eastern Lunatic Asylum in Williamsburg, Virginia. Over the next two centuries, mental health care took on various forms, but its leaders were almost exclusively psychiatrists (Feldman, 1981, p. 4). By the 1960s, with the federal emphasis on community mental health centers, administrators had begun to come from disciplines such as psychology, social work, and counseling (Feldman, 1981). The recent concern about having competent administrators in the public mental health system certainly was foreshadowed in 1971 when Hirschowitz addressed concerns over burnout and ineffectiveness among community mental health directors. He described the difficulty faced by clinicians who took on leadership roles as the "clinician-to-executive dilemma" (Hirschowitz, 1971, p. 102) and further mentioned how clinicians struggled to learn the skills necessary to be effective executive directors of community mental health centers. His concern was for the typical "trial by fire" (p. 104) that directors experience in their transition to administration. Hirschowitz (1971) believed that the successful leader would be "inspired by his ideology but must be guided by his knowledge of political strategy" (p. 104). He described the "armamentarium" (p. 104) of an effective clinician-turned-administrator as needing to include administrative, managerial, negotiating, political, and promotional skills, and he predicted that without these skills the leader would face a "navigator crisis" (p. 104).

Feldman (1973) has suggested that nine areas characterize the modern mental health services setting. These areas are

1. increased scope and resources,
2. larger and more diverse staffs,
3. complex organizational patterns,
4. multiple funding sources,
5. multi-unit systems coordinated with other services,
6. sophisticated management information and evaluation,
7. close involvement with government at all levels,
8. greater community involvement, and
9. increased sensitivity to change (pp. xiii–xiv).

In 1979, the National Task Force on Mental Health/Mental Retardation Administration, citing Feldman, stated, "To the clinician not trained in mental health administration, these characteristics pose difficult if not overwhelming barriers to the successful management of a mental health services system" (*Report*, 1979, pp. xiii–xiv).

Over the last few decades, mental health literature has pondered the type of training that will lead to more effective agency leadership. Feldman (1981) asserted that the successful community mental health administrator for the 1980s would be characterized by "a sense of humor, honesty, a high tolerance for ambiguity and frustration, the ability to anticipate the unintended effects of decisions, a distrust of power, and an irreverence toward the things that most people take too seriously" (p. 12). He also highlighted the need for administrative skills and an understanding of "what it is like to be a patient" (pp. 12–13). This discussion continued into the 1990s when Grusky, Thompson, and Tillipman (1991) debated whether a clinical background or a pure administrative background is best for mental health leadership. Those authors pointed out the value and necessity of both. Sluyter's (1995) research findings pointed out that state directors of mental health believe that more training in leadership and management is needed. This dialogue regarding the best training for mental health agency directors highlights the reality that, although clinical training benefits people in that role, it does not prepare an individual for the rigors and demands of an administrative job.

More recently, based on early work by Burns (1978), the discussion of what it takes to be an effective mental health administrator has emphasized the ideas seen in "transformational leadership." Corrigan, Garman, Lam, and Leary (1998) found that mental health workers wanted leaders who were less autocratic, dealt with problems in the organization, presented clear goals, fostered employees to find a higher meaning from their work, and effectively managed diversity. Corrigan, Diwan, Campion, and Rashid (2002) expressed the need for mental health agencies to manifest transformational leadership in order to decrease turnover and burnout rates among staff. Keshavan (2011), in discussing the need for global mental health leadership, has written that the mental health leader of the future "will need a combination of collaborative style, teaching ability, strong advocacy, communication, networking and systems coordination skills, apart from a realistic, persistent optimism" (p. 161).

The challenges and needs of mental health leadership are no different today than they were in the past. Ohio's community mental health agency directors work in an industry with high regulatory demands, narrow-to-no financial margins, high staff turnover, rapidly changing reimbursement structures, and extremely high service demands. The Associate Director of The Ohio Council of Behavioral Health & Family Services Providers has expressed concern that over the next five years many of the directors of community mental health agencies will be retiring. She has stated that because the field is so difficult leadership often falls to the "last counselor standing" (T. Lampl, personal conversation, October 2009).

Because of this looming loss of experienced leaders, it is extremely important that an effort be made to understand the unique developmental process of mental health directors in Ohio and to develop a support and mentoring structure to ensure good leadership at the agency level in the future. My hope is that this research study will provide salient information to aid executive directors. My findings may provide some of the necessary pieces and parts of such a mentoring or training program.

Significance of the Study

This study represents an endeavor to add to the current knowledge-base and increase the understanding of leadership development in Ohio's community mental health system. My intent was to gain insight into how community mental health center (CMHC) executive directors perceive their development as leaders and to identify the most effective ways of learning how to foster that development. Understanding this phenomenon may help others working to develop inexperienced or new mental health agency directors into effective leaders gain insight into the process involved in the maturation of the leaders-in-training. Specifically, understanding how successful mental health agency leaders have learned to do their job will provide insight into the kinds of activities or experiences that are needed to train new leaders. These insights also may be helpful in crafting a leadership training model for future CMHC executive directors.

Methodological Overview

The central purpose of this study was to gain an understanding of the developmental experiences of CMHC executive directors in Ohio who began their careers as clinicians. Because the focus of the study was to be able to describe the lived experience of the individuals as they move from the role of clinician into that of executive director and their growth process as administrators, the study drew on phenomenological research.

Research Questions

This study was guided by one primary question and three sub-questions. The primary question was, What is the developmental experience of CMHC directors who begin their careers as clinicians and become effective executive directors? The three sub-questions were as follows: (a) What do CMHC directors describe as the most helpful resources during this transitional process? (b) What are the most important lessons those directors have learned through those resources? (c) What competencies do the directors consider to be most important for them to learn? The reason for focusing on those four questions was to create an understanding of how successful directors have matured in their careers.

Theoretical Frame

The frame, or "worldview" (Creswell, 2007, p. 19), for this study was social constructivism. Guba and Lincoln (1994) defined the use of a constructivist paradigm as seeking to understand and describe the participants' experiences (p. 112). Creswell (2007) described the use of this paradigm as appropriate when research is focused on views and meanings of the situation (p. 20). Guba and Lincoln (1994) asserted that the aim of a constructivist's research is to understand and reconstruct the experience of another. The nature of knowledge in the constructivist paradigm, those authors said, is determined by how individuals reconstruct their experience of the topic, and knowledge accumulation is through vicarious experience (p. 112). For Guba and Lincoln, the intent of the constructivist paradigm was to give meaning to participant experiences. My aim by using this paradigm was, through providing increased understanding, to have a positive impact on future leadership development practices.

Adult learning theory was the first theoretical base, or frame, for this study. Allen (2007) has discussed the importance of adult learning theory as a foundation for leadership development. A second theoretical frame for my study was adult development. The idea that people develop throughout their lifetime has become an established concept in psychological literature (e.g., Birren & Birren, 1990). Maslow (1943), Erikson (1963, 1964, 1968), Kohlberg (1963), and Gilligan (1982) all described ways in which adult development occurs throughout a person's lifetime. These ideas are further developed in Chapter II of the present study.

Access

The Associate Director of The Ohio Council of Behavioral Health & Family Services Providers was used as the gatekeeper to help choose the people making up the sample for this study. The gatekeeper has a relationship with all of the members of the Ohio Council and is in a position to identify those who meet the following criteria: They have at least six years in transition from clinician to director in which to be able to identify their own development, and they are able to self-reflect and verbalize the experience and discuss its impact on themselves. The gatekeeper identified a pool of 10 subjects and, after reviewing the group for their ability to provide an intense description of the phenomenon, selected six for me to interview. Data analysis followed the method suggested by Creswell (2007) for phenomenological studies: I described my own experience; listened to the subjects, extracted salient and consistent themes; and have written a description of the phenomenon. An understanding of the forthcoming discussion requires familiarity with several special terms. In the next brief section, terms that are important to this study will be defined to clarify their specific meaning to this project.

Definition of Terms

Phenomenological inquiry: A type of inquiry in which the researcher is focused on understanding a particular experience or phenomenon. The researcher typically interviews subjects who have experienced the phenomenon and then organizes the information and data gathered from the interviews in a way that is descriptive of the essence of the lived experience.

Clinician: A mental health professional who works directly with patients to help ameliorate their mental health symptoms. Mental health professionals may come from any of several disciplines, including psychiatry, psychology, nursing, social work, or counseling.

Community Mental Health Center (CMHC): According to the federal government's Centers for Medicare and Medicaid Services (n.d.), a CMHC

    a. is an entity that meets applicable licensing or certification requirements for CMHCs in the State in which it is located; and

    b. must provide all of the following core services to meet the statutory definition of a CMHC....

    c. may receive Medicare reimbursement for partial hospitalization services only if it demonstrates that it provides such services. The core services include:

- outpatient services, including specialized outpatient services for children, the elderly, individuals who are chronically mentally ill, and residents of the CMHC's mental health service area who have been discharged from inpatient treatment at a mental health facility;
- 24-hour-a-day emergency care services;
- day treatment, or other partial hospitalization services, or psychosocial rehabilitation services; and
- screening for patients being considered for admission to State mental health facilities to determine the appropriateness of such admission (Section: "Survey and Certification, Certification and Compliance"; Chapter: "Community Mental Health Centers").

Executive director: An individual hired by the CMHC's board of directors who is responsible for all aspects of carrying out the agency's mission.

Developmental process: The maturational progression leaders go through as they experience their jobs and which leads them to understand their jobs better, lead better, and overall become better leaders and better people.

The Ohio Council of Behavioral Health & Family Services Providers: The trade association for community mental health centers in Ohio.

Experiences: Incidents that executive directors encounter as they lead; these may include relationships, successes, failures, conflicts, or challenges.

Resources: Any tool, be it a person, book, class, conference, practice, or discipline, that helps a leader develop, learn, and grow more effective.

Aspect [of a director's job]: Any part, responsibility, or requirement of the job.

Limitations and Delimitations of the Study

A researcher can control some elements of research but has little control over others. In relation to such control, Dusick (2011a) discussed the concept of assumptions and limitations within a research project. *Assumptions*, she reported, are "those things we take for granted in a study: statements by the researcher that certain elements of the research are to be understood to be true" (p. 1). According to Dusick (2011a), the theory under investigation, the phenomenon being studied, the methodology, the participants, and the results are all areas in which assumptions are made (p. 1). She further instructed that "elements [within a study] over which the researcher has no control" (p. 1) are known as the *limitations*. After defining assumptions and limitations, she laid out the connection between the two: Limitations often include (a) the researcher's assumptions, (b) how well the sample represents the population studied, and (c) how well the theoretical foundation of the study actually reflects the phenomenon studied (Dusick, 2011a, p. 1). Because it is important that the researcher clearly document any limitations that characterize the study, I followed Dusick to identify my assumptions, how well my sample represented the population, and whether my theoretical framework measured what this study is purported to investigate.

First, within this study, I made several assumptions that may have limited the genuineness of the results: I assumed that moving from the role of a clinician to that of an executive director involved a process of learning and developing; I assumed that effective leaders go through a never-ending process of learning how to be more effective at their jobs; and I further assumed that many directors are able to verbalize and describe this growth process. Second, in regard to how well the sample I used represents the population I studied, my study was confined to a select few executive directors who are working in the community mental health system in Ohio, and I will not be able to generalize the results to the broader population of leadership development. Third, in regard to the theoretical framework of adult learning theory and adult development, these theories may have limitations in being able to provide the constructs necessary to describe and capture the essence of the phenomenon of the leadership development experience for the executive directors I interview. Finally, because I, like the participants in this study, am an executive director of a mental health center who began my career as a clinician, I may find that I over identify with the participants and project my own thoughts and feelings into the research results. This limitation will be discussed in more detail in the reflections section of Chapter V.

Delimitations are the elements in a study that the researcher controls and uses to set the boundaries of the study. Delimitations include (a) the inclusion and exclusion of participants, (b) the instrumentation, and (c) the generalizability of the results (Dusick, 2011b, p. 1). In this present study, I specifically researched the experience of executive directors in Ohio's community mental health system that began their careers as clinicians and moved into these executive jobs; the study does not include executive directors with nonclinical backgrounds or directors outside of Ohio's community mental health system. The focus of the study was to describe the experience the directors had as they developed in their jobs. Because of this specific focus on experiences, I used a phenomenological approach: Subject interviews were the primary instrument involved in gathering data, and the data therefore was descriptive rather than quantifiable. This study focused on Ohio's community mental health directors who began their careers as clinicians. No other types of leaders were studied.

Summary

Mental health leadership is a very arduous vocation and yet is necessary in order to provide a competent network of care to those in our society who need it most. Over the years, researchers in the field have debated what type of training or background helps produce the most effective mental health administrators. Leaders who not only have a clinical background but also are trained in management and administration are identified as having a greater chance to be successful. The need to develop good mental health leadership is important in general, but in Ohio many of the current agency directors are known to be near retirement, making the understanding of how to facilitate the growth of such leaders even more pressing.

This present study seeks to use a phenomenological research approach to gain an in-depth understanding of the process of leadership development within community mental health centers in Ohio. Particularly, this project was targeted on understanding the development of individuals who enter the mental health field as clinicians and move into executive director positions at community mental health centers. A social constructivist paradigm framed the study because the prevailing assumption regarding how knowledge is acquired was that it is constructed via the experience of the subjects moving from the role of clinician to that of director.

My particular interest in this topic was fueled by both my work over the last 13 years in Ohio's community mental health system and the impact that the developmental process of becoming an effective leader has had on me. The sample used in this study was executive directors of Ohio community mental health centers who began their careers as clinicians. A total of six experienced directors were interviewed in order to explore the phenomenon of their development as leaders. It is my hope that the results of this study will assist the leadership of Ohio's mental health system in finding ways to support the development of effective leadership within its mental health community. The next chapter in this study is a review of literature. To better understand the concepts of how an adult experiences learning and development, along with how, in particular, leaders develop, I am presenting literature that delves not only into mental health leadership but into leadership in general. Areas of literature that were explored to provide a foundation for the study include adult development, adult learning theory, and personal growth and change.

CHAPTER II

Review of Literature

This study was an investigation of the experience of leadership development in executive directors of community mental health centers. It specifically sought to analyze the developmental process of executive directors who began their careers as clinicians. The study assumed that the experience of leading offers an opportunity for development toward being a more effective leader. It also assumed that adults in leadership roles can use the experiences, relationships, and events they encounter to help them understand themselves, their organizations, and the working relationships in which they engage, in a much more complex and meaningful way. I wrote this study through the paradigm, or framework, of social constructivism. The method I used was phenomenology. I chose phenomenology as my approach so that the clinician-to-leader experience can be captured in the voice of the participants; their stories may be helpful in assisting others traveling the same path in the field of mental health agency leadership.

I began to investigate the process of mental health leadership development by examining two bodies of literature, social constructivism and phenomenological research. After presenting research exploring these two components of my dissertation, I explored literature to support the study. To fully develop the idea that there is a developmental process among mental health leaders, I have established the framework for the research by exploring several concepts that relate to mental health leadership, leadership in general, learning, adult development, and personal change.

Phenomenology and Constructivism

The phenomenological approach used in this study was a qualitative method. The approach was birthed out of Husserl's (1970) philosophical ideas that one's life experiences shape and form one's reality or interpretations of life. Merriam (2009) said that Husserl's philosophy of phenomenology underlies all qualitative research. The underlying concept in phenomenological philosophy, claimed Merriam, was that how one experiences life events becomes the conscious reality of that experience (p. 24). In other words, people define reality or truth based on their experiences with it. For example, if several educators were to describe what being a teacher is like, they would each most likely give a different description. Each would have had a different experience, and therefore their realties may be subtly or starkly different.

Phenomenological studies explore the nature and meaning of experience (Van Manen, 1990). A phenomenological study, therefore, according to Van Manen (1990), asks the question, What is this or that kind of experience like? (p. 9). Phenomenological research is often called the study of a *lived experience* (Patton, 2002 p. 104), and Van

Manen (1990) described that brand of research as the study of essences and of experiential meanings as they are lived, the explication of phenomena as they present to one's consciousness, and thus the search for what it means to be human (pp. 9–12). Merriam (2009) has stated that "the task of the phenomenologist, then, is to depict the essence or basic structure of experience" (p. 25). In view of that task, the phenomenological researcher relies often on interviews of participants who have experienced a phenomenon being studied. This type of research requires researchers to explore their own experiences with the phenomenon and to become aware of their own biases, opinions, and assumptions regarding the subject. Researchers therefore must work at setting aside their personal biases and viewpoints in order to understand the subject in a more pure way. Such suspension of bias is known as the *epoche* of phenomenological research (Moustakas, 1994, p. 33).

Moustakas (1994) stated that in phenomenological research perception is regarded as the primary source of knowledge. He went on to describe the nine core principles that embody this type of inquiry: (a) focusing on the appearance of things; (b) having a concern for "wholeness"; (c) finding the essence of the appearance through intuition and reflection; (d) describing the subject matter rather than analyzing it; (e) researching from a position of personal interest that focuses on the meaning of the experience; (f) integrating the subject and the object; (g) keeping in mind that both intersubjective reality and researcher perception are part of the process; (h) remembering that the researcher's intuition, reflection, and judging are the primary evidence for investigation; and (i) ensuring that the question being researched is very carefully and deliberately constructed (closely paraphrased from Moustakas, 1994, pp. 52–59).

Because the paradigm for this project was social constructivism, the purpose of my study was to use data from the research participants to identify and define the process of developmental growth that they have experienced as clinicians becoming directors of mental health centers. The participants were asked to identify events, experiences, resources, and relationships from which they have learned and how those factors helped them develop as leaders. According to Creswell (2007), this type of question, the description of an experience, emanates from a "worldview" (p. 19) of social constructivism. Guba and Lincoln (1994) said that a constructivist paradigm seeks to correctly interpret and describe the participant's experience (p. 112). Creswell (2007) has described the use of this paradigm as appropriate when research is focused on views and meanings of a particular situation (p. 20). Guba and Lincoln (1994) also stated that the aim of constructivist's research is to understand and reconstruct the meaning of another person's experience. The nature of knowledge within this paradigm, they claimed, is the individual reconstruction of the topic and the accumulation of knowledge through vicarious experience (p. 112). Using Guba and Lincoln's ideas, this study sought to give meaning to the participants' experiences and to frame those experiences as leadership development.

Researchers who approach their work from a constructivist paradigm are operating from the foundation that what is considered objective knowledge or truth comes from one's perspective on the subject (Schwandt, 1994, p. 125). Schwandt (1994) mentioned that Nelson Goodman was the first philosopher to define the constructivist theory. Goodman (1984) said that reality or "versions" come from how one perceives or constructs what one sees and experiences (p. 35). Guba and Lincoln (2005) pointed out that the paradigm of social constructivism is posited on various practical issues in research. They asserted that the overall aim of inquiry within constructionism is to gain understanding and to reconstruct a meaning for the subject, and they noted that the nature of the understanding comes from a collective reconstruction built upon consensus of the research participants as passionate participants (Guba & Lincoln, 2005, p. 194). Ontologically, they contended, constructivism centers on a participative reality, the "subjective-objective reality cocreated by the mind and given cosmos" (p. 195). In other works, Guba and Lincoln (1989, 2001) described what distinguishes the constructivist paradigm from other systems used for research or inquiry. They also stated that constructivism's three basic assumptions are what provide the primary distinction. Ontologically, then, constructivism is based on relativism (Guba & Lincoln, 2001, p. 1). These researchers pointed out that the use of relativism does not mean "anything goes" (2001, p. 1), but that traditional concepts used to determine truth and accuracy, such as validity, reliability, and objectivity, are not relevant. Instead, they maintained, the ideas of credibility, transferability, dependability, and confirmability are appropriate. They described credibility as being

> roughly parallel to internal validity, established by prolonged engagement at the site, persistent observation, peer debriefing (a kind of external critic), negative case analysis (a process of reworking postulated hypotheses), progressive subjectivity (continuous checking of developing constructions against records of constructions that were expected prior to data collection), and (most important) member checks, continuous testing of hypotheses, data, preliminary categories, and interpretations with members of stakeholding audiences. (Guba & Lincoln, 2001, p. 13)

These authors went on to describe transferability as similar to external validity, established by the researchers having their descriptions of the topic confirmed by others reading and evaluating their interpretation (Guba & Lincoln, 2001, p. 13). Dependability, Guba and Lincoln (2001) added, relates to reliability, being determined through an outside evaluator assessing the methodological decisions that were made and the reason for those decisions (p. 14). Finally, they related confirmability to objectivity. This method of evaluation, they said, relates to an outside evaluator assessing "the extent to which constructions, assertions, facts, and data can be traced to their sources" (p. 14).

Defining Leadership Development

Mental Health Leadership—Administrative versus Clinical Training

Having defined phenomenology and social constructivism, the next sections explore the topic of leadership development. I begin by reviewing and analyzing research related to leadership in the field of mental health. In the field of mental health leadership, I discuss development in two ways, beginning with the body of literature concerned with developing administrators for clinics and hospitals and concluding with the literature related to development of clinical supervisors. Austin (1991) discussed the need for more effective training in mental health demonstration in terms of matching what students learn to what they actually do on the job. He presented a three-step process in which a clinician or therapist moves from being a clinician to being an administrator, with the steps being (a) clinician to supervisor, (b) supervisor to program director, and (c) program director to executive director (Austin, 1991, pp. 234–235).

Developing administrators for community mental health organizations. Perlman and Hartman (1987) pointed out the need for management training for mental health administrators for community mental health agencies but mentioned that few, if any, programs of that type existed. They asserted that training in "systems knowledge" (p. 40) is most important and suggested that the American Psychological Association develop courses for new managers. Grusky, Thompson, and Tillipman (1991) stated that little research had been done concerning the preferred background for mental health leaders. They compared and contrasted the benefit of a clinical versus an administrative background in relation to what makes the better mental health administrator. They felt that the clinical background lends itself to working with staff and other managers but concluded that much of what is required in mental health leadership is administrative. Thus they considered as ideal a comprehensive approach to background and training that incorporates both clinical and administrative training (Grusky et al., 1991, p. 277). Sluyter's (1995) study of 45 state mental health directors regarding their beliefs about what types of training are needed in mental health administration indicated that more training in leadership and management was needed, with training for supervisors of direct service staff rated first, followed by the need for training of senior administrators (p. 203).

Corrigan, Garman, Lam, and Leary (1998) researched the type of leadership qualities that frustrated staff in mental health clinics. Their research led to the conclusion that staff members were frustrated with supervisors whose leadership style was controlling, who had difficulty making decisions, and who did not foster teamwork or make work meaningful. Workers preferred a leader who operated from a transformational paradigm, one who could help give them a sense of personal accomplishment from their work and foster a positive organizational culture. Corrigan, Diwan, Campion, and Rashid

(2002) found that transformational leadership had a positive impact on the mental health treatment team. Workers longed for leaders who could help them make their work personally meaningful, inspire teamwork, and decrease burnout. The information related to the training of mental health administrators is paralleled to some degree by research focused on developing clinical supervisors. Research related to counselor development has led to similar studies about supervisory development. The next section will present literature related to the development of clinical supervisors.

Developing clinical supervisors. The second thread of literature involving leadership development in the field of mental health addresses the development of clinical supervisors. Watkins (1990) identified four stages of development for a psychotherapy supervisor. He reported that fully developed supervisors are characterized as having (a) confidence in their skill, (b) insight regarding their impact on supervisees, (c) an approach to supervision that is based on theory, and (d) a strong sense of professional identity (p. 555). Baker, Exum, and Tyler (2002), studying the Watkins model as it related to clinical supervisors in training, found that as supervisors gained more experience their confidence grew. Nelson, Oliver, and Capps (2006) also studied the development of doctoral students as clinical supervisors. Those researchers found six themes emerging as a developmental process for supervisors: "learning," "supervisee growth," "individual uniqueness," "reflection," "connections," and "putting it all together." Barnes and Moon (2006), also studying the Watkins model, found that it was demonstrably reflective of supervisor psychological development.

The studies specifically exploring mental health leadership development help set the larger stage for understanding the developmental process that mental health administrators might go through. To further clarify the meaning of leadership, the following section reviews the basic tasks of leadership and also identify the type of leadership that the mental health literature identifies as important for the field.

Basic Tasks and Types of Leadership

Leadership has many definitions. The theories about how a person leads range from the concept that leadership skills are innate in some individuals and not in others to the belief that leadership is a set of skills that anyone can learn. Northouse (2010) has discussed the leading approaches and theories in leadership, which range from trait-based and skill-based approaches to modern theories such as transformational leadership and authentic leadership. Trait-based leadership theories, also known as "great man theories," focus on the concept that leadership abilities are innate, great leaders are born that way, and only great people possess such traits (p. 15). Skill-based approaches to leadership theory move away from the focus on personality and innate abilities and promote the idea that leadership is a set of skills that can be taught to and learned by others (p. 39). Transformational leadership theory is based on the concept that leaders can change, bring out the best in, and inspire followers. This theory integrates "charismatic and visionary leadership" into how the leader impacts others (p. 171). According to Northouse, authentic leadership is one of the "newest areas in leadership research" and focuses on the "authenticity" or genuineness of a leader's behavior (p. 205). Each of these theories represents an aspect of leadership and may help demonstrate how multifaceted leadership is as a concept.

Amit, Popper, Gal, Mamane-Levy, and Lisak (2009) saw a vacuum in research focused on the use of comprehensive methodological discussion in the developmental psychological aspects of leadership development. They reported that research has traditionally focused on outstanding leaders and a psychoanalytic viewpoint of leaders' development, and they stated that leadership research overall has been concerned primarily with how "leadership as an independent variable affects followers' attitudinal and performance variable" (p. 303). In an effort to help fill this vacuum, I explored research from a different perspective than the one that Amit et al. reported as predominant in the literature: I investigated how the experience of leading generates change and development. To discuss how leaders develop, however, I must begin with an exploration of the concept of leadership. For my study, leadership is defined through the concepts developed by Burns (1978); Gardner (1990); Drath and Palus (1994); Luthans and Avolio (2003); Avolio and Gardner (2005); Gardner, Avolio, Luthans, May, and Walumbwa (2005); and Walumbwa, Avolio, Gardner, Wernsing, and Peterson (2008).

Gardner's functional definition of leadership. Gardner (1990) identified the tasks of leadership that in essence can serve as his functional definition of being a leader. The first task he identified was *envisioning goals*; he believed that leaders accomplish the task of setting goals in diverse ways and that goals "emerge from many sources" (p. 12). Some leaders' goals are handed to them by higher authorities, he said, but other leaders may spend lengthy time with their constituents establishing common goals. The second task of leadership, according to Gardner, is *affirming values*. He pointed out that society is held together by shared values but that "values always decay over time" (p. 13) and that, because of this decay, "There must be perpetual rebuilding" (p. 13). Gardner stated, "Societies that keep their values alive do so not by escaping the process of decay, but by powerful processes of regeneration" (p. 13). Because of this cycle of decay, he felt that a task of leadership is to pilot the revitalization of the shared values. Gardner's third task for leadership is *motivating*. He claimed that leaders do not create motivation but rather "unlock or channel existing motives" (p. 14), and he observed that each group has a "tangle of motives" (p. 14). The effective leader, he asserted, is one who can draw on the motives that provoke others to action around shared goals. Effective leaders also confront issues that keep others from giving their best. In the end, he said, "they [effective leaders] create a climate in which there is pride in making significant contributions to shared goals" (p. 14).

The fourth task Gardner (1990) identified was *managing*. He made it clear that there is a difference between leading and managing but also said that the two categories "overlap" (p. 14). The components of leading that he categorized as managing are planning and priority, organizing and institution building, keeping the system functioning, agenda-setting and decision-making, and exercising political judgment (pp. 15–16). The fifth task of leadership for Gardner was *achieving workable unity*. He stated that "all leaders must spend part of their time dealing with polarization and building community" (p. 17) and he emphasized trust as a key component to accomplishing that undertaking. Another leadership task Gardner listed was *explaining*. Although he admitted that this role may be seen as "too pedestrian" (p. 17), he explained that "every leader recognized it" (p. 17) as being part of what they do. He believed that those who can explain well will find themselves leading, even if they are not in leadership roles. *Serving as a symbol* was an additional task of leadership identified by Gardner. Along with that symbolic task, he felt, goes the task of *representing the group*. Finally, Gardner said that leaders have the task of *renewing*. He admitted that some leaders may not be "renewers" (p. 21) but affirmed that renewal nonetheless is an important aspect of what is needed by followers.

Leadership as transformational. Gardner's work helps clarify the specific details of the work done by leaders. As he described the work done by leaders, he identified concepts such as envisioning, fostering unity, and renewing. Burns (1978) also looked at the behavior of leaders. He developed the idea that leadership brings out the very best in followers. Burns distinguished between leadership that is transactional and leadership that is transformational. He began by describing leadership as an aspect of power. "Leadership over human beings," he said, "is exercised when persons with certain motives and purposes mobilize, in competition or conflict with others, institutional, political, psychological, and other resources so as to arouse, engage, and satisfy the motives of followers" (Burns, 1978, p. 18). Burns distinguished between leaders and "power wielders" (p. 18) by clarifying that "[a]ll leaders are actual or potential power holders, but not all power holders are leaders" (p. 18). He advocated seeing power and leadership not as things but as relationships.

Burns (1978) defined leadership as "inducing followers to act for certain goals that represent the values and motivations—the wants and needs, the aspirations and expectations—of both leaders and followers" (p. 19). Transactional leadership, he said, involves the exchange of "valued things" (p. 19): It is a relationship in which each party is getting something for themselves out of the relationship and the goals pursued are not shared. In view of Sergiovanni's (2007) work (for example, pp. 78–79), this relationship can be considered to be a coercive type of leading. Burns (1978) described transformational leadership as occurring "when one or more persons engage with others in such a way that leaders and followers raise one another to higher levels of motivation and morality" (p. 20) and further defined it as being concerned with end values such as liberty, justice, and equality (p. 426). Leaders who are driven by such higher-level values or motivators, he indicated in reference to Maslow (1943), can only pursue those leadership goals once they have moved through other levels of motivation (Burns, 1978, pp. 65–67). Burns (1978) then went on to describe how people who have achieved Maslow's highest level of psychological need, "self-actualization," are potential leaders. Burns stated, "[T]he concept of self-actualization is a powerful one for understanding the process of leadership" (p. 117). He said, in regard to how self-actualization relates to the development of leaders, "I suggest the most marked characteristic of self-actualizers as potential leaders goes well beyond Maslow's self-actualization: It is their capacity to *learn* from others and from their environment—the capacity *to be taught"* (p. 117; italics in original). Burns then defined self-actualization in leadership development by stating that it is *"to lead by being led"* (p. 117; italics in original).

Bass (1985) described transformational leadership as raising the consciousness of shared goals, helping team members move past their own self-interest for the good of the team, and motivating others toward higher-level needs. Bass and Avolio (1990) listed four distinguishing factors of transformational leadership: idealized influence (charisma), inspirational motivation, intellectual stimulation, and individualized consideration (p. 248). "Idealized influence" in their model refers to leaders being compelling role models for those they are leading. Leaders practicing idealized influence demonstrate high morals and ethics in their behavior; they offer a keen sense of mission and vision for followers and are highly respected. "Inspirational motivation" refers to leaders expecting a lot from their followers and inspiring those followers to be devoted to the organization's shared vision. "Intellectual stimulation" describes leaders who foster followers' creativity, encouraging them to be inventive and celebrating innovation. "Individualized consideration" refers to the leadership behavior of listening and supporting followers. Transformational leaders thus seek to assist their followers in becoming self-actualized. Such leaders seek to treat their followers individually and hence provide various styles of interaction. For some followers, transformational leaders will be directive, whereas for others they may allow more freedom.

Leadership as "meaning making." Both Burns (1978) and Gardner (1990) discussed leadership at its best as a force that develops individuals, teams, and organizations. They envisioned leaders who encourage the uniting of individuals and groups around higher values. These types of leaders also unify individuals and groups around a common organizational vision and mission. Drath and Palus (1994) viewed leadership much the same way but took the concept a step further by depicting leadership as creating meaning for the followers. They described conceptualizing leadership as "meaning making" (p. 2) and contrasted five concepts in demonstrating the difference between leadership as meaning making and the traditional approach based on dominance. Their contrasts included seeing leadership as (a) creating "social meaning-making" versus imposing "social influence" (p. 14), (b) facilitating people's participation in a "shared process" (p. 14) versus empowering a "dominant individual leader" (p.14) to act on followers, (c) channeling people's intrinsic motivation versus assuming the need to provide external motivation (p. 17), (d) being an authority figure in a participative process of leadership versus being a leader because of one's authority (p. 18), and (e) participating in an effective process versus needing to take charge to get results (p. 19). The concepts described by Drath and Palus go beyond the idea of leaders imposing their will on others to accomplish a task. These authors challenged leaders to lift others up and to help them become better people by finding meaning and purpose in their work.

Authentic leadership. According to Northouse (2010), *authentic leadership* represents one of the latest themes in leadership research. The final view that framed my understanding of the meaning of leadership for the present project is the theory of authentic leadership as presented by Luthans and Avolio (2003), Avolio and Gardner (2005), Gardner et al. (2005), and Walumbwa et al. (2008). All these authors use a developmental approach to authentic leadership theory.

Luthans and Avolio (2003) defined the theoretical foundation of authentic leadership as coming from positive organizational behavior, transformational full-range leadership, and ethical leadership (pp. 245–250). They identified five positive characteristics that frame the behavior of an authentic leader, describing authentic leaders as (a) guided by a set of end values that represent an orientation toward doing what is right for their constituency; (b) operating with no gap between espoused values and values in action; (c) remaining cognizant of their own vulnerabilities and openly discussing them with associates so the leader can be questioned to ensure that the direction they are heading is "right"; (d) using actions characterized as "walking the talk" (p. 248), by leading from the front while modeling hope, confidence, optimism, and resiliency; and (e) having developed the moral capacity to judge issues and dilemmas that are characterized by "shades of gray." Increased self-awareness in turn regulates behavior and leads to authentic leadership behavior, described by Luthans and Avolio, in table format, as "confident, hopeful, optimistic, resilient, transparent, moral/ethical, future-oriented, and associate building" (p. 251).

In defining authentic leadership, Avolio and Gardner (2005) stated that it "can incorporate transformational, charismatic, servant, spiritual, or other forms of positive leadership" (p. 329). Gardner et al. (2005) discussed authentic leadership as encompassing "authentic relations with followers and associates [that] are characterized by: (a) transparency, openness, and trust, (b) guidance toward worthy objects, and (c) an emphasis on follower development" (p. 345). Walumbwa et al. (2008) defined authentic leadership as "a pattern of leader behavior that draws upon and promotes both positive psychological capacities and a positive ethical climate to foster greater self-awareness, an internalized moral perspective, balanced processing of information, and relational transparency on the part of leaders working with followers, fostering positive self-development" (p. 94). Luthans and Avolio (2003), Avolio and Gardner (2005), Gardner et al. (2005), and Walumbwa et al. (2008) all identified a model for authentic leadership development. Their combined description emphasized that authentic leadership is a process of development that occurs as the leader begins with positive psychological capabilities, in a positive organizational context, then experiences trigger events or challenges that lead to increased self-awareness.

The theoretical frameworks of Burns (1978), Gardner (1990), and Drath and Palus (1994), along with the theory of authentic leadership, as defined above, shaped how leadership was understood in my research. These authors all view leadership skills, abilities, and behaviors as elements that change as a leader goes forward in his or her life. Their theories provide a framework to measure leaders as they grow and develop their skills over time. The concept of adults experiencing psychological, social, and moral growth and development throughout their lifetimes was developed by Maslow (1943), Erikson (1964, 1968), Kohlberg (1969), and Gilligan (1982), whose work suggests a developmental course that moves toward a more moral, ethical, and authentic person. The work of all of these researchers on adult development provides an important foundation to undergird the idea of leaders developing over the course of their careers.

The Role of Adult Development in Leadership Development

The idea that people develop throughout their lifetimes has become an established concept in psychological literature (Birren & Birren, 1990, pp. 8–10). A number of models describe how adults develop throughout life. For the purposes of this study, four theorists will be used: Maslow (1943), Erikson (1963, 1964, 1968), Kohlberg (1963, 1976), and Gilligan (1982) each expressed ideas about how adult development occurs throughout one's lifetime. They conceptualized the movement toward a more ethical, selfless, and moral state of being. Maslow (1943) is important because of his concept of adults being able to reach "self-actualization" (p. 382). Erikson (1963) described adults as being able to move into "generativity" (p. 266), with the adult's focus on giving and helping others. Kohlberg (1976) described moral development as being able to reach a point where "universal ethical principles" (p. 35) are the motivating factors in an adult's behavior. Gilligan (1982) described how women develop morally based on an "ethic of care" (p. 74). Each of these concepts is critical for leaders to be able to be transformational and authentic and to make meaning for their followers as they lead.

Maslow's theory of self-actualization. Maslow's (1943) developmental model, described as a hierarchy, identifies the primary motivators that drive human behavior. He explained that people move from pursuing the most basic human needs, which he called *survival needs*, all the way up to what he considered the highest need, known as *self-actualization*. He explained that at this highest level a human being is "doing what he is fitted for" (p. 7). Maslow conceptualized that these levels of motivators are actually developmentally progressive and form a hierarchy. Individuals, he felt, cannot move into the next higher level of motivation until they have satisfied their previous and current level of motivation.

Maslow (1943) also described human beings as being in a constant state of "wanting" (p. 12). He asserted that such a state of wanting seeks, at the lowest level, to meet physiological needs (p. 2). According to Maslow, physiological needs include such things as water, nutrition, and oxygen. After these are met, people are driven by safety needs (p. 4), the pursuit to live in a safe environment that provides peace and stability. Maslow's third level of need is the need for love and affection (p. 6). At this level, he said, individuals are motivated to find friendship and emotionally close relationships. The next motivation for Maslow, once individuals' love needs are met, is for self-esteem (p. 6). At that level, people pursue a "stable, firmly based (usually) high evaluation of themselves for self-respect, for self-esteem, and for the self-esteem of others" (p. 6). Maslow's final and highest level of motivation, the need for self-actualization, is the need that manifests itself when all other needs are thoroughly satisfied:

> Even if all other of these needs are satisfied, we may still (if not always) expect that a new discontent and restlessness will soon develop, unless the individual is doing what he is fitted for. A musician must make music, an artist must paint, a poet must write, if he is to be ultimately happy. What a man can be, he must be. This need we may call self-actualization. (Maslow, 1943, p. 382)

Maslow believed that satisfied people were rare; therefore this final stage remained "a challenging problem for research" (p. 383).

Maslow's (1943) hierarchy of needs theory seems to point to the prospect that people have the capacity to strive toward selflessness, contentedness, and a highly meaningful level of being. When applied to leadership development, these concepts allow for leaders to stretch and grow into a more authentic or transformational form of leadership. Maslow's concept of self-actualization, "doing what one is fitted for," could easily be used to describe the genuineness of an authentic leader.

Erikson's concept of generativity. Just as Maslow's (1943) theory provided a way to look at adult development as a series of levels, Erikson (1963) proposed a series of developmental crises that individuals must resolve in order to accomplish emotional development successfully. Erikson asserted that people grow and develop emotionally until death in a series of eight psychosocial stages (1963, pp. 247–274). The strength of

Erikson's theory is in helping human development to be understood as a continuum of psychosocial stages (Hamachek, 1990, p. 677). Although Erikson's theory applies to the entire life span, his ideas that are included in the sixth, seventh, and eighth stages describe the profile of an adult who has experienced positive development. Similarly to Maslow's concept of self-actualization, Erikson's (1964) seventh stage, generativity, refers to successful development for an adult between the ages of 35 and retirement from work. The characteristics of the generative adult help lay a foundation for describing the type of leadership discussed earlier through the work of Burns (1978), Gardner (1990), Drath and Palus (1994), Luthans and Avolio (2003), Avolio and Gardner (2005), Gardner et al. (2005), and Walumbwa et al. (2008).

The first five of Erikson's (1964) stages – trust versus mistrust, autonomy versus shame and doubt, initiative versus guilt, industry versus inferiority, and identity versus role confusion — are stages that people encounter in the first 19 years of life. The last three stages span the rest of adulthood. Stage 6, intimacy versus isolation, occurs during early adulthood, from ages 19 to 24. During that stage, the primary concern is finding love and intimacy with others. The eighth and final stage, integrity versus despair, is experienced in the retirement years as individuals seek to validate their life experience and end their days with a sense of meaning (Boeree, 2006), but it is the seventh stage that holds the most importance for my research into leadership development.

Erickson's (1964) seventh stage, generativity versus stagnation, which adults experience from ages 25 to 64, represents a time when an individual can transition into a person capable of being a leader who reflects a transforming and meaning-making style and who is authentic in his or her approach to leading. Bradley and Marcia (1998) identified the main task of the seventh stage as guiding the next generation with acts of care. They believed that the two basic components of generativity are *involvement* and *inclusivity*. Adults who have fully developed into generative people, they said, display both of these components: A generative adult is highly involved in the work and growth of young people and is also concerned with the broader societal issues, tolerant of different ideas, and able to balance caring for self and caring for others (p. 42). Another look at generativity comes from McAdams and de St. Aubin (1992), who described a generative person as ready to make a commitment to the larger sphere of society and to seek its continuation and improvement through the next generation. Those researchers stated that a person can be generative in a variety of life pursuits, including professional activities and volunteerism (p. 1003). Based on their view, generativity can be seen in the way one leads an organization.

Erikson (1968) wrote that his theory of development follows the epigenetic principle, concerning which he said, "[A]nything that grows has a ground plan, and ... out of this ground plan parts arise, each part having its time of special ascendency until all parts have arisen to form a functioning whole" (p. 92). Erikson also believed that each psychosocial crisis would manifest itself throughout lives and personalities: "For man, to remain psychologically alive, must resolve these conflicts unceasingly, even as his body must unceasingly combat the encroachment of physical decomposition" (1959, p. 51). Kotre (1984) broadened the definition of generativity. He wrote "generativity may be defined as a desire to invest one's substance in forms of life and work that will outlive the self" (p. 10). He felt that generativity could be differentiated into four types: biological, parental, technical, and cultural (p. 12). In biological generativity the object focused on is a new-born infant. The actions of this type of generativity are "begetting, bearing, and nursing offspring" (p. 12). Parental generativity refers to being focused on one's child and includes the actions of "nurturing and discipline one's offspring, [and] initiating them into a family's traditions" (p. 12). Kotre described technical generativity as being "accomplished by teachers at all stations of the journey through life, who pass on skills to those less advanced than themselves" (p. 13). Here the action is on "Teaching skills—'the body' of a culture—to successors, implicitly passing on the symbol system in which the skills are imbedded" (p. 12). The fourth type of generativity, cultural, is "directly concerned with mind" (p. 14). The action is on "[c]reating, renovating, and conserving a symbol system…" (p. 12). Here the teacher is "no longer a teacher of skills but a mentor, and her apprentice has become a disciple" (p. 14).

Kotre (1984) explained the concept of generativity as having four distinct types. Hamachek (1990) further described those who have fully developed the trait of generativity as concerned for others, focused more on giving than on receiving, absorbed in activities outside of themselves, wanting to be productive and contribute to society, displaying "other-centered values," wanting to enhance what is known even if it means changing the status quo, and wanting to develop their talents and express themselves uniquely (p. 679).

Erikson asserted that although eight primary stages manifested themselves at definable times of life, each of the eight are present at all ages and surface within the context of the primary crisis (Slater, 2003, p. 54). Slater (2003) expanded on Erikson's ideas and contended that the stage of generativity versus stagnation manifests throughout each phase of a person's life. He named the six phases leading up to generativity as inclusivity versus exclusivity, pride versus embarrassment, responsibility versus ambivalence, career productivity versus inadequacy, parenthood versus self-absorption, and being needed versus alienation (pp. 60–63).

Kohlberg's and Gilligan's concepts of moral development. Complementing the theories of Maslow and Erikson, Kohlberg (1963, 1976) and Gilligan (1982) both proposed that people begin a developmental process in childhood that can continue into adult life. Their work centered on moral development. Kohlberg (1976) proposed that "to understand moral stage [sic] it is helpful to locate it in a sequence of development of personality. We know that individuals pass through the moral stages one step at a time as they progress from bottom (Stage 1) to top (Stage 6)" (p. 31). He conceived six stages of moral development that fall into three major levels and theorized that individuals progress through the stages horizontally as they develop the intellectual capacity to think more abstractly, and vertically as they move from more self-focused morality to a morality centered on universal ethical principles (Kohlberg, 1963, p. 9).

At Kohlberg's (1976) most basic level (Stage 1), individuals are focused on "heteronomous morality" (p. 34). At this stage, they are motivated to do right simply to avoid punishment. Stage 2 represents "individualism," where rules are followed in order to "serve one's own needs" (p. 34). In Kohlberg's Stage 3, individuals do right in order to meet the expectations of others, function cognitively at the conventional stage, and have internalized the rules and expectations of others, whereas at Stage 4 they do right in order to keep society going as a whole (pp. 33–35). Stages 5 and 6 in Kohlberg's hierarchy represent the stages at which individuals have chosen the principles in life by which they want to live and are able to think at the most abstract levels. At Stage 5, the society's social contract or utility and individual rights are the motivation; at Stage 6, what Kohlberg called "universal ethical principles" (p. 35) become the primary motivation. It is at Stage 5, and more so at Stage 6, that leaders who are practicing transformational or authentic leadership practices evolve. In order to lead in such a way as to increase the unity of their constituents, make meaning, and grow in an authentic leadership style, individuals must hold fast to Kohlberg's higher levels of moral development, including the appreciation of individual rights and, most importantly, of universal ethical principles.

Gilligan (1982) challenged Kohlberg's (1976) theory as being insufficient to describe the moral development of females. She stated that Kohlberg's theory of moral development is "based empirically on a study of eighty-four boys whose development Kohlberg has followed for a period of over twenty years" (Gilligan, 1982, p. 18). She expressed concern that groups not part of the sample in his study "… rarely reach his higher stages" (p. 18) and went on to say that "the very traits that traditionally have defined the 'goodness' of women, their care for and sensitivity to the needs of others, are those that mark them as deficient in moral development" (p. 18). Out of her concern for the inadequacy of Kohlberg's theory to address the moral development of females, Gilligan put forward her own theory. Her belief was that, rather than their moral development being rooted in "rights," as she stated was Kohlberg's construction, women structure morality around "responsibility" to others (p. 19). She contended, "In this [her own] conception, the moral problem arises from conflicting responsibilities rather than from competing rights and requires for its resolution a mode of thinking that is contextual and narrative rather than formal and abstract" (p. 19). She believed that for women a moral construct based on responsibility focused on "connection" to others, rather than "separation" from others, was the reality (p. 19).

Gilligan (1982) stated that her concept of moral development manifested itself in terms of an "ethic of care" (p. 74). She asserted that in the initial stage of moral development females make moral decisions based on "caring for the self in order to ensure survival (p. 74). As a woman progresses through this orientation, according to Gilligan, she becomes increasingly concerned with her responsibility to others and moves into the second phase of development, in which "good is equated with caring for others" (p. 74). In the third and final phase of moral development, Gilligan saw "a shift in concern from goodness to truth" (p. 82). In this phase, she said, a woman begins to ask "if it is possible to be responsible to herself as well as to others" (p. 82) and starts to consider if it is possible for her to make moral decisions based on a concern for both self and others.

The Role of Learning in Leadership Development

The theories of Maslow (1943), Erikson (1963, 1964, 1968), Kohlberg (1963, 1976), and Gilligan (1982) laid the groundwork for the principle that adults develop psychologically, socially, and morally over their lifetimes. According to these authors, development occurs in an adaptive pattern, causing individuals to grow more self-actualized in their desires for life, more generative in their approach to life, and more focused on universal ethical principles in their view of morality. As people develop, then, it is important to also establish how processing and learning from their experiences facilitate that development. Also, because leaders can be assumed to change their behavior over the course of their leadership life, based on learning, it is important to understand how researchers believe learning happens. Piaget and Inhelder (1969), Bronfenbrenner (1979, 1989), and Bandura (2004) each presented a theoretical model that will support an understanding of how learning from experience takes place.

Cognitive development theory. The cognitive development theory of Piaget and Inhelder (1969) laid the groundwork for understanding learning by identifying four factors that lead to cognitive development (pp. 154–157). The first is "organic growth and especially maturation of the nervous system" (p. 154). The second is "exercise and the acquired experience in the actions performed upon objects" (p. 155). Webb (1980), in describing this second factor, explained how experience relates to learning. She said that "experience ... aids in discovery of the properties of objects and in the development of organizational skills" (p. 93). Piaget and Inhelder's (1969) third factor is "social interaction and transmission" (p. 156). They stated that this factor is "necessary and essential" (p. 156), but that it is "insufficient by itself" (p. 156). They discussed the need for the learner to be an active part of the reception and "assimilation" and said that the "individual contributes as much as he receives" (p. 156). Their final factor, identified as necessary for cognitive skill development, they called "self-regulation" and linked to maintaining an "equilibrium" or a "series of active compensations ... in response to external disturbances" (p. 157). That final factor, they said, involves the process in which individuals take in new information and adapt their current understanding to incorporate the new information.

Piaget and Inhelder's (1969) theory of learning describes how the bits and pieces of data are absorbed into a person's mind and transformed into useful knowledge. They called the constructs of information that are grouped together to form how people understand or give meaning to the life around them "schemes" (p. 4). Schemes, they claimed, fit together and make up the basic understanding one has of life. As long as these schemes are not challenged by new or conflicting information, Piaget and Inhelder asserted, there is a balance in understanding life as it is going on around an individual. They believed that as people come into contact with information or experiences that challenge the scheme, a process must occur to manage the new data, and people have two options for dealing with the new information: They can either assimilate it, meaning add it to the existing scheme, or accommodate to it (Piaget & Inhelder, 1969, pp. 5–6). For them, accommodating to new feedback meant actually changing one's scheme to adapt to the old one or creating a new scheme that would adjust to the new reality.

Piaget and Inhelder's (1969) work provides the mechanism and terminology necessary to understand the basic processes involved in learning. As leaders experience new information during the tenure of their leadership, they are likely to experience information that challenges the schemes with which they are operating. Leaders then either add this new information to their existing scheme or adapt by changing their existing scheme or creating a new one. If one were to lay Piaget and Inhelder's process parallel to the developmental ideas of Maslow (1943), Erikson (1963, 1964, 1968), Gilligan (1982), and Kohlberg (1963, 1969, 1976), it is possible to see how the work of schemes through assimilation and accommodation assists in adult development. In addition to Piaget and Inhelder (1969), Bronfenbrenner (1979, 1989) and Bandura (2004) have added complexity to the mechanism of how information and feedback from the environment cause learning and changes in behavior.

Social learning theory. Bandura's (2004) social learning theory provides another perspective on how adults adapt their behavior through learning, insight, and development of understanding. Bandura maintained that adults adapt behavior based on their environmental experiences and on "behavior, cognitive, and other personal factors" (p. 27). He used the term *triadic reciprocality* first to make clear that human behavior is not simply driven individually, by either environmental or internal characteristics, but that both characteristics simultaneously affect human behavior, and second to assert that behavior, environmental factors, and personal factors all impact one another in a "bidirectional" fashion (p. 27). According to Bandura, applying the concept of triadic reciprocality to how leaders develop during the course of their leadership experience demonstrates clearly that the environment and the personal traits of leaders impact their growth. At the same time, the behavior of leaders impacts and shapes the environment and the team that surround them. This bidirectional influence, said Bandura, creates a dynamic process that allows both the leaders to shape their environment and the environment to shape the leaders. By recognizing the impact the environment has on their development, then, leaders can reflect and analyze their experiences to help improve and adapt their skills. Believing that this self-reflective ability was what set humans apart, Bandura (2004) stated,

> If there is any characteristic that is distinctively human it is the capability for reflection and self-consciousness. This enables people to analyze their experiences and to think about their own thought process. By reflecting on their varied experiences and on what they know, they can derive generic knowledge about themselves and the world around them. People not only gain understanding through reflection, they evaluate and alter their own thinking. (p. 40)

Bandura (2004) theorized that people learn about adapting their behavior through four sources of information: "performance attainments; vicarious experiences of observing the performances of others; verbal persuasion and allied types of social influences that one possesses certain capabilities [*sic*]; and physiological states from which people partly judge their capabilities, strength, and vulnerability" (p. 41). As individuals experience these four factors, he said, they make choices about what they can and should do. Leaders, as they lead, encounter success, failure, challenges, victories, and defeats. Each of these becomes a filter through which the leader can choose to adapt in the next circumstance. Bandura's theory provides an added complexity to learning when laid over Piaget and Inhelder's ideas. It provides a way for leaders to facilitate their development by reflecting on how they are using the four types of feedback they receive.

Ecological systems theory. Bronfenbrenner (1979, 1989; see also Bronfenbrenner, Kessel, Kessen, & White, 1986) explored the depth to which individuals' thoughts and behaviors are impacted by the highly complex and interwoven systems in which they live. He developed the ecological systems theory to describe the complexities out of which human behavioral choices grow and also proposed that all of a person's "biological, cognitive, emotional, and social elements are intertwined" (Bronfenbrenner et al., 1986, p. 1223). Bronfenbrenner also developed an elaborate model that describes the interaction among the many systems in an individual's life. In that model, he identified five levels at which people live and are influenced: The first is the *microsystem* (Bronfenbrenner, 1979, p. 7). Bronfenbrenner (1979) defined the microsystem as "a pattern of activities, roles, and interpersonal relations experienced by the developing persons in a given setting with particular physical and material characteristics" (p. 22). He gave examples of what he meant as a setting to include one's home, a child's playground, or where there are "face-to-face interactions" (p. 22). The next layer, the *mesosystem*, is essentially "a system of microsystems," he said (p. 25): For example, individuals' lives and choices are impacted by how their roles at home and work interact. Problems or stressors experienced in a person's role as boss at the work place can have an influence or impact on his or her mood at home and hence affect his or her role as spouse or parent. Bronfenbrenner (1979) asserted that within the mesosystem of adults, work conditions have a dramatic effect on how one functions as a spouse and a parent (p. 236).

The third layer in Bronfenbrenner's (1979) model is the *exosystem*, which is made up of systems in which individuals do not participate, but that nonetheless impact them. Decisions made by groups within the exosystem impact an individual's behavior both directly and indirectly. Bronfenbrenner cited examples of a child's exosystem as "the parent's place of work, a school class attended by an older sibling, the parents' network of friends, the activities of the school board, and so on" (p. 25). Bronfenbrenner's fourth system, the *macrosystem*, consists of the shared beliefs and values around which groups are organized. He defined it as "consistencies, in the form and context of the lower ordered systems (micro-, meso-, and exo-), that exist, or could exist, at the level of the subculture or the culture as a whole, along with any belief systems or ideology underlying such systems" (p. 26). Lemme (2006), in referring to Bronfenbrenner's model, described the macrosystem as including "social classes, ethnic groups, or even entire societies" (p. 43). The paradigms, religions, political systems, and other pervasive beliefs at this systemic level shape the ideas through which behavioral choices are made, according to Bronfenbrenner(1979). The final system, which was identified by Bronfenbrenner in a later work (1989), is the *chronosystem*, the dimension of time. He referred to the chronosystem as related to "developmental changes triggered by life events or experiences" (p. 201) and went on to say that "these experiences may have their origins either in the external environment … or within the organism" (p. 201). Further describing the events and experiences in the chronosystem, Bronfenbrenner said, "Whatever their origin, the critical feature of such events is that they alter the existing relation between person and environment, thus creating a dynamic that may instigate developmental change" (p. 201).

Bronfenbrenner's theory (1979, 1989; see also Bronfenbrenner et al., 1986) can be helpful to leaders as they examine the various influences that affect their decision-making and behavioral choices. Understanding these systems and how the systems influence their behavior may assist leaders in making more informed choices regarding how they interact with others and with their surroundings.

Learning by Leading

The previous section of this literature review presented information related to how theorists believe learning and behavioral change occur. I used the theories of Maslow (1943), Erikson (1963, 1964, 1968), Kohlberg (1963, 1976), Gilligan (1982), Piaget and Inhelder (1969), Bandura (2004), and Bronfenbrenner (1979, 1989; see also Bronfenbrenner et al., 1986) to explain how various factors related to one's life experience, environment, and relationships lead to behavior change and learning. That information provides an essential foundation as this study now begins to analyze how leaders describe their experience of learning and developing on the job. First, in this section learning is described in both its simple and more evolved form. Next, I investigate the theories that apply learning to leadership development.

The most effective leaders view learning as a critical element to their effectiveness. Johnson (2008) has stated,

> Effective leaders are effective not because they have more knowledge or experience than ineffective leaders; but rather, it is because they have a more valid and effective way of handling the complex issues they face. The difference between effective and ineffective leaders is their mental models or meaning structures, the way they handle and deal with their world. (p. 85)

Learning through one's leadership experience can be simply informational, as in learning the best way to put together a schedule to make sure there is good shift coverage, or transformational, in which a leader learns that rather than focusing on the schedule itself, the real source for a good work schedule is workers who are motivated to do the work and so finds ways to align the mission of the job with what the employees find meaningful. Kegan (2000) contrasted informational and transformative learning. He described informational learning as useful for increasing one's bank of knowledge or for increasing skills, expanding already existing cognitive capabilities into new areas, whereas he considered transformative learning as involved in changing not only *what* one knows but *how* one knows (pp. 48–49).

Models that describe the process of how people change through the process of learning include Bateson's (1972) four levels of learning; Watzlawick, Weakland, and Fisch's (1974) second-order change; and Argyris and Schön's (1974) double-loop learning. Bateson's theory of learning introduces the concept of transformative learning, and it is important to look at his ideas first in this next section because they lay the foundation for both double-loop learning and second-order change (Hawkins, 2004, p. 410).

Learning as a Process of Change

Bateson's four levels of change. Bateson (1972) defined learning as a process of change, saying, "The word 'learning' undoubtedly denotes *change* of some kind. *To what kind of change is a delicate matter*" (p. 283; italics in original). He believed that all "biological and evolving systems (i.e., individual organisms, animal and human societies, ecosystems, and the like)" were made up of "cybernetic networks" (p. 447), and he described these cybernetic networks as large systems made up of subsystems, all of which were self-correcting. Within the context of this belief, Bateson hypothesized four levels of learning. He believed that each level of learning was necessary and potentially used by human beings. Similar to Maslow's (1943) idea of a hierarchy of needs, Bateson's learning levels build on one another; in other words, a person cannot learn at level three without having first learned at level zero. The first level, *zero learning,* is described by Bateson (1972) as "the simple receipt of information from an external event in such a way that a similar event at a later (and appropriate) time will convey the same information" (p. 284). Minimal change occurs in the state of zero learning (Bale, 1992, referring to Bateson). Bateson, as related by Bale, gives an example of a laborer learning that the whistle blowing means it is twelve o'clock. This type of learning does not contain a trial-and-error component, but two types of errors can be made. If the context offers two alternatives, a person could either correctly employ the information that signals these alternatives but choose the wrong alternative or misidentify the context and choose the wrong alternative (Bale, 1992, pp. 16–17).

Bateson (1972) referred to the second level of learning as *learning I.* Learning I refers to what is commonly known as "trial-and-error learning, instrumental learning, or conditioning" (Bale, 1992, p. 17, referring to Bateson). Bateson (1972) succinctly defined learning I as "change in the specificity of response by correction of errors of choice within a set of alternatives" (p. 293). He described the difference between this and zero learning as "changes in zero learning" (p. 287). For learning I and any other type of learning to take place, he said, there must be repeatable contexts (p. 288). Bateson gave examples of learning I as applying various behaviors in different contexts, such as those of boxers shaking hands at the beginning of a fight and then proceeding to fight, the different responses for an air-raid siren and an all-clear siren, and various observances of etiquette. This type of learning is described by Watzlawick et al. (1974) as *first-order change* and by Argyris and Schön (1974) as *single-loop learning.*

The next level, *learning II,* was characterized by Bateson (1972) as "change in the process of learning, e.g., a corrective set of alternatives from which choice is made, or ... a change in how the sequence of experience is punctuated" (p. 293). This level of learning, Bateson felt, reflects the "unconscious phenomenon wherein we learn about and classify the context in which learning takes place" (Bale, 1992, p. 19, referring to Bateson). During level II learning, individuals no longer allow themselves to be bound by the alternatives learned for the context in which the learning occurred but now are able to consider other options. Bale suggested that this is how musicians learn to play the same instrument but adopt various styles, such as classical or folk or rock (p. 19). Tosey (2006) described learning II as being "essentially about the pattern of context in which activity takes place." (p. 7). The awareness of the context and of making nontraditional (non-level I) choices is the idea seen in the second-order-change theory pioneered by Watzlawick et al. (1974). Tosey (2006) considered the application of level II learning in management and organizational context as reframing how one views politics as "metarules for context" (p. 8) rather than seeing them as negative.

Level III learning, the fourth level, was identified by Bateson (1972) as "a change in the process of learning II, e.g., a corrective change in the system of sets of alternatives from which the choice is made" (p. 293). Bateson believed that learning III was a rare phenomenon and that most human beings do not have, or ever gain, the capacity for it. Individuals are triggered to reach this level of learning when they experience "contraries" (p. 305) to their learning II commitments, Bateson believed, and he considered learning III a dangerous territory that could lead to psychosis. Bateson believed that level three, when it is achieved by humans, leads to forgetting oneself:

> If I stop at the level of Learning II I am aggregate of those characteristics which I call my "character." I am my habits of acting in context in which I act. Selfhood is a product or aggregate of Learning II. To the degree a man achieves Learning III, and learns to perceive and act in the terms of contexts of contexts his "self" will take on irrelevance. The concept of "self" will no longer function as a nodal argument in the punctuation of experience. (Bateson, 1972, p. 304)

Bateson's (1972) four levels of learning provide a basic structure for understanding transformative learning. To further explore the concept of how learning can be transformative, I will next review the work of Watzlawick et al. (1974) on the concept of second-order change.

First- and second-order change. As part of their jobs, leaders will experience a variety of situations and circumstances to which they must adapt. Based on the traditional learning theories of Piaget and Inhelder (1969) and of Bateson (1972), most leaders will learn to do their tasks based on trial and error. Their experiences will be organized into various "frameworks or schemata" (Bartunek & Moch, 1987, p. 484). The concept of first- and second-order change provides a way to conceptualize how learning can be categorized as either "informational or transformative" (Kegan, 2000). First-order changes are changes or adaptations based on the current established way of understanding, whereas second-order changes involve modifying the established framework (Bartunek & Moch, 1987; Watzlawick et al., 1974). Second-order change requires people to actually modify their basic beliefs and perceptions (Evans, 1996, p. 17).

When operating from a paradigm within first-order change, persons must learn to adapt their behavior based on the solutions offered within the system in which they work. The changes or adjustments made are made within the existing structure or system; no new learning is required, and the change is not transformational. Essentially, the problem or challenge is viewed the same way and, essentially, the same types of interventions are continually applied. When second-order changes are applied, they create a new solution that is designed to change the system. Second-order changes are transformational: They involve changing the system or paradigm, they require new knowledge and skills, they break with the past, and they disrupt homeostasis (Bateson, 1972; Bergquist, 1993; Buker, 2003; Waters, Marzano, & McNulty, 2003; Watzlawick et al., 1974).

Single- and double-loop learning. Akin to the ideas of first- and second-order change is the notion of single- and double-loop learning. As with the two types of change discussed above, these two levels of learning describe stages of growth in a person's understanding of the deeply complex relationships, problems, and challenges found in working and leading.

Leadership in organizations involves problem-solving. Based on the prior research on learning (Bandura, 1977, 2004; Piaget & Inhelder, 1969), the types of solutions that are applied to problems stem from how a leader understands the situation and what he or she has learned about such problems. The terms *single-loop* and *double-loop learning* differentiate the varying levels of complexity or depth by which a leader views and intervenes. Argyris (1991) expressed concern that most leaders define problems too narrowly and fail to be reflective about how they are defining issues. When leaders are not reflective, they are likely to not consider how their own perspectives perpetuate the problem.

Single-loop learning is characterized by focusing on the problem through the lenses of the existing paradigm, system, or definition. During single-loop learning, actions and strategies are sought, but the basic governing principles, assumptions about the situation, or beliefs about the circumstances are not challenged (Allen, 2001, p. 9); that is, the prevailing goals and objectives are not questioned (Foldy & Creed, 1999, p. 213). Argyris and Schön (1974) proposed that managers and leaders in organizations typically engage in what they called "single-loop learning," which they described as problem-solving in which the values and presuppositions involved with the problem are not questioned.

Double-loop learning, a concept also first proposed by Argyris and Schön (1974), distinguishes between two types of problem-solving done by individuals and organizations. When persons engage in double-loop learning, they begin to question the underlying beliefs about the problem. The authors gave the following example:

> When the error detected and corrected permits the organization to carry on its present policies or achieve its present objectives, then that error-and-correction process is single-loop learning. Single-loop learning is like a thermostat that learns when it is too hot or too cold and turns the heat on or off. The thermostat can perform this task because it can receive information (the temperature of the room) and take corrective action. Double-loop learning occurs when error is detected and corrected in ways that involve the modification of an organization's underlying norms, policies, and objectives. (Argyris and Schön, 1974, pp. 2–3)

In double-loop learning, leaders change their values (Foldy & Creed, 1999, p. 208), which results in the assumptions and beliefs about the situation being challenged (Allen, 2001).

Bateson's (1972) four levels of learning, Watzlawick et al.'s (1974) second-order change, and Argyris and Schön's (1974) double-loop learning all describe the mechanisms at work in leadership development. Their theories provide a vehicle for understanding how leaders change through complex ways of processing their experience. In the final section of this literature review, I present researchers who have developed specific models to describe the process of change that leaders experience as they develop.

The Change Process and Leadership Development

Quinn, Spreitzer, and Brown (2000) made the statement, "Change does not come easily" (p. 147). Although this may be an understatement, it is also likely true that development and change as a leader do not come easily. The previous sections of this literature review have developed the concepts that form the foundation of adult development and learning. In this final segment, I will discuss the theories of Amey (2005); McKenna, Yost, and Boyd (2007); Bennis and Thomas (2002); Goleman, Boyatzis, and McKee (2002); and Quinn et al. (2000) as a way to explore how adult learning, growth, and development specifically apply to leadership.

The cognitive process model. The concept that leaders do not just emerge but go through a cognitively based learning and developmental process was discussed by Amey (2005). She stated that "leadership involves cognitive processes, meaning-making for self and others, and has a developmental orientation" (p. 690). Amey went on to say that leadership "constructed as learning looks as though it develops along a developmental continuum" (p. 695). She presented a model of leadership development that occurs in three stages, during which the leader moves from a "top-down orientation" to finally becoming more "servant-like," "relationship oriented," and focused on "cocreating meaning" (p. 696).

Specifically, Amey (2005) suggested that in the first stage of development leaders view their job from a top-down orientation. The primary characteristics of their behavior are focused on being the single leader, conflict negotiator, and primary communicator; thus they are focused on task accomplishment and set the mission and direction. In Amey's Stage 2 as experience forces change in the leaders' cognitive schema for their jobs, they begin to view leadership from a facilitative and inclusive orientation. Their behavioral characteristics move toward being more participatory and toward flattening the hierarchy; their focus is more on establishing a learning environment and fostering shared goals while still accomplishing tasks than on individual employee task accomplishment: There has been a turn to group goals. Overall, these leaders increasingly move toward involving others in decision-making. By the third stage of learning and development in Amey's model, the leaders have moved into the servant-like leadership orientation. Their behavior has become that of "guide," "facilitator of processes," and "translator" (p. 696). Their focus is on relationships and on cultivating an ongoing culture of learning for their employees. The groups and teams have become "self-governing" and "interdependent," and the leaders have begun "cocreating meaning" for themselves and the others (p. 696).

Amey's (2005) model provides a construct to view the change that occurs as leaders assimilate and accommodate to new information. The model demonstrates how environment and personal characteristics interact to help a leader become more servant-like. Thus, viewed through the lens of Bronfenbrenner (1979, 1989), one can say that the systems in a leader's life shape his or her learning and behavior and provide a way to view leadership learning as a developmental process.

The work experience model. Researchers over the last several years have suggested that work experience is the place a great deal of learning and development occurs for leaders (Bennis & Thomas, 2002; McCall, Lombardo, & Morrison, 1988; McKenna, Boyd, & Yost, 2007; McKenna, Yost, & Boyd, 2007; Robinson & Wick, 1992). A specific example is found among religious leaders: McKenna, Yost, and Boyd (2007) studied clergy leaders and concluded from their study that

> there are a predictable set of lessons that pastors learn in their leadership journeys. These lessons are in the areas of handling relationships, managerial thinking, personal and ministerial values, personal awareness, and God's role in their lives. (p. 187)

Their study of 100 clergy leaders showed that 32% of the leadership "development experiences occurred in the trenches," (p. 179), 27% occurred in "times of transition," and 23% were within "personal relationships" (p. 179). McKenna, Boyd, and Yost (2007) learned that "there is considerable overlap with the situational factors and personal strategies important for business executive leadership development although significant differences were evident as well" (p. 198). They found that a key to leadership learning was personal reflection on what the leaders could learn from their experiences. They also found that using the feedback from others who could be reflective with the pastors and help the pastors process the experience was useful. The authors encouraged pastors to be intentional about their learning and to view each challenge as an opportunity to "strengthen their faith and prepare for the next leadership opportunity" (p. 200).

Similarly to McKenna, Yost, and Boyd (2007), Bennis and Thomas (2002) described leadership learning and development as occurring in "the crucibles of leadership" (p. 87). These authors stated, "[W]e have identified the process that allows an individual to undergo testing and to emerge, not just stronger, but equipped with the tools he or she needs both to lead and to learn" (Bennis & Thomas, 2002, p. 4). One of the core elements of their model is that leaders use their experiences to help themselves develop key leadership competencies. The four competencies Bennis and Thomas identified were "adaptive capacity, engaging others by creating shared meaning, voice, and integrity" (p. 89). They described adaptive capacity as being the "key" (p. 91). *Adaptive capacity*, in their view, includes the qualities of hardiness, learning skills, and creativity. *Shared meaning making*, they asserted, includes the practice of seeking out differing and dissenting opinions from which to learn. *Voice* to them meant having a strong sense of self-awareness, and *integrity* referred to a leader's having a moral compass. Each of these four competencies and their components were described by the authors as being developed over time and honed through the crucible experiences.

The self-directed learning model. Goleman et al. (2002) believed that the "crux of leadership development is self-directed learning" (p. 109). Boyatzis (1999) described an approach related to finding the discontinuity between one's "real self" and one's "ideal self" (p. 18). Goleman et al. (2002) outlined the process by identifying five discoveries that lead to the development of the ideal self as a leader (pp. 111–112). Their theory centers on learners first identifying their *ideal* self. This discovery of the ideal self is about taking time to process and envision the persons and leaders that they want to be. The second discovery is the *real* self, for which learners take an honest inventory of how they currently see themselves in comparison to their ideal selves. The third discovery is to develop a learning agenda, which is done only after learners have identified the strengths they possess and the gaps between their real and ideal selves. The fourth discovery involves experimenting with new behaviors, thoughts, and feelings; and the fifth discovery is to develop trusting relationships that support each stage of the process. Practicing these new behaviors, claimed Goleman et al., leads the learner to the discovery of the ideal self.

The advanced change model. Quinn et al. (2000) proposed a 10-point leadership change model, named the "Advanced Change Theory" (p. 148), which is an outline for how leaders can develop into more authentic or transformational leaders. The first phase of the model involves having a leader who seeks to create an emergent system; they described this leader as one who strives for inclusion, openness, and development while minimizing the need for hierarchy (p. 150). In the second phase of the Advanced Change Theory (ACT) model, the leader recognizes hypocrisy or patterns of self-deception (p. 151). In fact, Quinn et al. commented on the congruence of their ACT model with the ideas of Argyris (1991), who stated that human beings tend to organize their lives around remaining in control, winning, suppressing negative feelings, and making a rational pursuit of objectives. The third step in the ACT model is "personal change through value clarification and alignment of behaviors" (Quinn et al., 2000, p. 151), meaning that the leaders examine themselves for "self-hypocrisy" (p. 151). The model then encourages leaders to "free themselves from external sanctions," (p. 152), no longer worrying about public opinion. Next, the leaders must develop a vision for the common good. As they move forward, the leaders gain great courage and act on faith, taking themselves beyond the safe and conventional options; Quinn et al. described this stage as being on the "edge of chaos" (p. 153). Those authors went on to describe the transformation as including a "reverence of others involved in the change" and as "inspiring others to enact their best selves" (pp. 153–154). The developing leader, they asserted, "models counterintuitive and paradoxical behavior" (p. 155); finally, they said, leaders following the ACT model find that they have changed not only themselves but also the system in which they work. As Quinn et al. explained the ACT model they frequently referred to Gandhi and Jesus Christ as leaders who had demonstrated their model.

Summary

The purpose of this research study was to examine and describe the leadership development experience of community mental health center executive directors who began their careers as clinicians. In this chapter, I have provided a review of the scholarly literature relevant to the study. I began by laying the foundation of the paradigm and methodology used for the study. The paradigm through which the study is formed is social constructivism. Guba and Lincoln (1989, 1994, 2001, 2005) were used to define social constructivism and to discuss its application in research. This study was conducted using a phenomenological approach. The work of Husserl (1970), Van Manen (1990), Moustakas (1994), and Merriam (2009) provided an overview of the nature, purpose, and meaning of a phenomenological study. After establishing the paradigm and theoretical approach in which framed the study, I presented literature in the key areas of research that will provide the foundation for the exploration of community mental health center executive director development.

In the section following constructivism and phenomenology, I have explored leadership development. First, the work of Gardner (1990) and his tasks of leadership were presented to provide a practical conceptualization of the day-to-day work required of leaders. Second, Burn's (1978) contrasting of transactional and transformational leadership was used to frame a definition of leadership as stimulating others to act out of internal motivation. Third, the work of Drath and Palus (1994), who conceptualized leadership as meaning making, was discussed in terms of how it further defines leadership as a means to elevate others to becoming their best selves. The work of Avolio and Gardner (2005), Gardner et al. (2005), and Walumbwa et al. (2008) and the theory of authentic leadership concluded this section by conceptualizing leadership development as it leads to self-awareness, genuineness, wisdom, and pro-constituency behavior.

After defining leadership development as it pertains to this project, I have presented the notion that adults grow and develop over the course of their lives. Theoretically, this idea of continual development is important because it underscores the concept that people newly established in leadership roles develop as they gain experience. In order to establish this developmental component, I have referred to Maslow's (1943) theory of motivating factors, Erikson's (1963, 1964, 1968) model of psychosocial stages, and Kohlberg's (1963, 1969, 1976) ideas regarding moral development.

Following the section on the foundation of leadership theory and adult development, I have investigated the idea that adults learn to change their behavior based on their experience. I then have used the work of Piaget and Inhelder (1969) and Bronfenbrenner (1979, 1989; see also Bronfenbrenner et al., 1986) to advance the idea that adults develop and learn in the context of the systems in their lives, and I have presented Bandura's (1977, 2004) social learning theory to offer the idea that human beings learn and adapt their behavior based on experience.

After exploring the concept that adults adapt their behavior based on experience, I have presented the work of scholars who clarify the idea that learning occurs at progressively more complex levels and that the most complex levels involve individuals beginning to change not only *what* they know but also *how* they know. I have discussed Bateson's (1972) levels of learning as a way to conceptualize that learning takes place on a continuum of simple to very complex and have presented the model of double-loop learning (Argyris & Schön, 1974) as a way to reinforce the notion of learning complexity. Finally, I have offered the second-order change model of Watzlawick et al. (1974) to provide a framework for understanding how reflexive learning can lead to changing and deeper levels of understanding.

The last major idea I have explored is that effective leadership involves personal change, growth, and development. I have used Quinn et al. (2000); Amey (2005); McKenna, Yost, and Boyd (2007); McKenna, Boyd, and Yost (2007); Bennis and Thomas (2002); and Goleman et al. (2002) to explore how leadership involves a development growth process.

The ideas, theories, and models presented in this literature review point out that people continue to develop emotionally, psychologically, and morally as they age. The research presented also indicated that people learn and change as they have new experiences throughout their lives. This study used these concepts to explore the evolutionary dimension of leadership of community mental health center directors, seeking to understand how top administrators can and do develop into leaders who are more reflective, moral, selfless, and transformational leaders.

CHAPTER III

Research Methodology

As was established in the previous chapter, the idea that there is a definable developmental course that leaders follow as they mature and become more effective has been explored and characterized by a number of authors, including Amey (2005); Goleman, Boyatzis, and McKee (2002); Bennis and Thomas (2002); and Quinn, Spreitzer, and Brown (2000). In addition, research in mental health leadership has explored the need for good administrative training (Austen, 1991; Corrigan, Diwan, Campion, & Rashid, 2002; Corrigan, Garman, Lam, & Leary, 1998; Grusky, Thompson, & Tillipman, 1991; Perlman & Hartman, 1987; Sluyter, 1995); however, recent research in the area of leadership development specific to the field is not abundant. Most of the current research has focused on the developmental process of clinical supervisors (Barnes & Moon, 2006; Nelson, Oliver, & Capps, 2006; Watkins, 1990) rather than on agency or organizational leadership. In order to add research in the area of mental health agency leadership, this study will explore the experience of development from clinician to executive.

I used the technique of interviewing to investigate the story of the participants' journeys as evolving leaders. Turner and Mavin (2008) reported that most of the mainstream leadership literature "does not make known the emotions, self-doubt and questioning, thoughts and feelings associated with becoming a leader" (p. 378). Understanding the emotional and self-questioning aspects of the journey was a salient factor as I attempted to understand the path of development for mental health executive directors who began their careers as clinicians. Thus my interviews sought out the ways in which events, experiences, and relationships have impacted each participant's transformation from clinician to director. The inquiry explored the emotions, thoughts, and questions the directors experienced as they evolved.

Methodology

Conceptual Frame

The conceptual frame for this project is identified here to clarify the values that influence the question, paradigm, theory, and context of the study. Glesne (2006) pointed out that all research is done with the values of the researcher influencing how the researcher approaches a topic. Lincoln and Guba (1985) introduced five corollaries to the role of values in qualitative research: First, they stated that the values of the researcher influence the choice of the problem to be studied, the evaluation methods, and the way the problem is framed. They then asserted that the values inherent within the research paradigm, the theoretical lens used for the study, and the values within the context of which the study occurs all influence the inquiry (pp. 38, 174–177). Those authors pointed out the necessity for congruence between the values that influence the researcher, the paradigm, the theory, and the context in order for the research to be meaningful (p. 38).

Lincoln and Guba (1985) strongly encouraged researchers to disclose their values or biases, thus giving their readers a perspective in which to judge the research (p. 176). Based on this notion, and in order for my research project to produce meaningful conclusions, In the following sentences I have identified the values that I believed influenced me during this study. A value that I have always held in high regard is personal growth. This value clearly influenced my choice of research question, as the project is centered around the growth and development of mental health agency leadership. I believe that the challenges and experiences of the job shape the leader and can be a learning tool for new leaders if they choose to be self-reflective about how their emotions, vulnerabilities, skills, perceptions, choices, and personality are impacting their leadership. My bias is that I believe effective leaders are reflective and open to criticism about how they practice and that they seek to learn from their successes as well as their failures. Another bias I hold is that good leaders strive to be authentic (Walumbwa, Avolio, Gardner, Wernsing, & Peterson, 2008) and transformational (Burns, 1978). Luthans and Avolio (2003) described several characteristics of authentic leaders: Such leaders, they said, (a) are guided by a set of end values that represent an orientation toward doing what is right for their constituency; (b) permit no gap between their espoused values and their values in action; (c) remain cognizant of their own vulnerabilities, openly discussing them with associates in order to be questioned and to ensure that the direction they are heading is "right"; (d) lead from the front and model hope, confidence, optimism, and resiliency; and, finally, (e) demonstrate the moral capacity to judge issues and dilemmas that are characterized by "shades of gray" (pp. 248–249).

Very much in sync with the theory of authentic leadership is the concept of transformational leaders, who guide their followers in such a way that they assist them in living at a higher level of ethical and value-based behavior. Burns (1978) described transformational leadership as leadership that leads followers to higher manifestations of morality and motivation (p. 20). He stated that in this type of leadership the relationship between leader and follower is based on "mutual support for a common purpose" (p. 20), and he further described it as a "moral" type of leadership that "raises the level of human conduct and ethical aspiration of both leader and led, and thus it has a transforming effect on both" (p. 20). Most important, he said, is that transformational leaders "address themselves to followers' wants, needs, and other motivations, as well as to their own, and thus they serve as *an independent force in changing the makeup of the followers' motive base through gratifying their motives"* (Burns, 1978, p. 20; italics in original).

Another value that influenced my approach was the belief that people make sense of their own lives and experiences by constructing their own meanings for and perceptions of those experiences. This value aligns with the constructivist paradigm that undergirds my study. The theories of adult development and adult learning that frame the study also align with the values that I hold concerning personal growth, behavioral change, and meaning-making that occur as adults experience life.

Paradigm and Theoretical Frame

The purpose of this study was to use data from the research participants to identify and define the process of developmental growth they have experienced beginning as clinicians and becoming directors of mental health centers. The participants were asked to identify events, experiences, resources, and relationships from which they have learned and to explain how those experiences helped them develop as leaders.

According to Creswell (2007), this type of question, the description of an experience, emanates from a "worldview" (p. 19) of social constructivism. Guba and Lincoln (1994) described the use of a constructivist paradigm as seeking to correctly interpret and describe the participant's experience (p. 112). Creswell (2007) considered this paradigm appropriate when research is focused on views and meanings of a particular situation (p. 20). Guba and Lincoln (1994) claimed the nature of knowledge within this paradigm is the individual reconstruction of the topic and the accumulation of knowledge through vicarious experience (p. 112). The intent is to give meaning to the participant's experiences and frame them as leadership development.

The present study has two theoretical frames: adult learning theory and adult development theory. These two concepts provide the background research and models needed to understand interview data through the lens of a process that occurs during the course of becoming a leader. Allen (2007) evaluated the importance of adult learning theory as a foundation for leadership development (p. 26). He described behaviorism, cognitivism, social learning theory, developmentalism/transformative learning, and transfer of learning as concepts within the theory of adult learning that apply to leadership development (pp. 27–34). Allen asserted that each of these perspectives helps describe aspects of how adults learn and change. Each theory, he said, explained how adults change using a different emphasis to explain how or why change occurs. He further stated that from the behaviorist's perspective, "thinking and feeling have little to do with learning because they cannot be measured" (Allen, 2007, p. 27). The focus of learning for behaviorists is on the here and now. According to Allen, learning for behaviorists is characterized by measurable behavioral changes that are outlined and planned before the learning takes place (p. 27), and a behaviorist approach involves establishing goals and objectives toward which the emerging learner can strive (p. 28).

After describing behaviorism, Allen (2007) described the theory of cognitivism. He believed that the Gestalt theory of psychology is the foundation for cognitivism and that it "focuses on the internal aspects of learning" (p. 29). Cognitivists, he said, believe that learning is a function of the interaction of persons and their environment (pp. 30–31). In other words, individuals have various experiences, they must assimilate that information into their current bank of knowledge and understanding, and so learning takes place as individuals adjust to this new information by adapting their perceptions, interpretations, and behaviors.

Another one of the concepts in adult learning theory that Allen (2007) felt applied to leadership development, social learning theory, suggests that learning occurs by observation of modeled behaviors (p. 31). Bandura (1977), the founder of social learning theory, believed that most learning takes place by observing others' successes or failures (p. 22). Allen (2007) discussed the importance of this concept in leadership development by encouraging leaders to understand their organizational culture and to be aware of the importance of the congruence between the behaviors that are modeled and the espoused beliefs of the organization (p. 32).

Allen's (2007) next application of adult learning theory to leadership development, developmentalism/transformative learning, reflects the idea that learning takes place by individuals reflecting on the meaning of their environment and experiences. Through reflection, individuals enlarge their current points of view, either by transforming their view or by changing their "habits of mind" (Allen, 2007, p. 33). The concept of self-awareness along with reflection and learning from prior actions and its importance to leadership development is seen in the work of Goleman et al. (2002), who discussed self-awareness as a key to leaders' acting with "conviction and authenticity" (p. 40).

The last option for adult learning mentioned by Allen (2007) is transfer of learning (p. 34). Transfer of learning relates to the experience of individuals' learning by internalizing information from training or educational opportunities and adapting their behavior accordingly (Caffarella, 2002, p. 204). Allen (2007) suggested that this option for leadership development is often underutilized yet important because when learning occurs it often does not transfer to work-related behaviors (p. 35).

The idea that people develop over the course of a lifetime has become an established concept in psychological literature (see, e.g., Birren & Birren, 1990). Erikson (1964, 1968), Gilligan (1982), Kohlberg (1963, 1969, 1976), and Maslow (1943) all described ways in which adult development occurs throughout one's lifetime. Based on the cited research, this project assumed that the subjects are learning from trial and error, gaining new ways of interpreting their experiences, listening to feedback, and growing more effective and authentic.

The worldview of social constructivism, along with the theories of adult learning and adult development, drove the methods used for this study. Interviewing was the primary tool used to gather data, and the purpose of the interviews was to elicit from the participants their description of how they have experienced their own leadership development. Specifically, the interview questions targeted the successes, failures, difficult decisions, challenges, mentors, feedback, and self-reflection that have informed and shaped the participants' leadership experiences.

Design

To effectively study the process that CMHC executive directors describe as their development into leaders, I used a phenomenological study. Phenomenological studies are utilized to explore the nature and meaning of experience (Van Manen, 1990). A phenomenological study asks the question, "What is this or that kind of experience like?" (Van Manen, 1990, p. 9), and thus it is often called the study of a *lived experience* (Creswell, 2007; Patton, 1990). Van Manen (1990) further described it as the study of essences, of experiential meanings as they are lived, the explication of phenomena as they present to one's consciousness, and the search for what it means to be human (pp. 9–12).

Moustakas (1994) stated that in phenomenological research, "perception is regarded as the primary source of knowledge" (p. 52). He went on to describe the core principles that embody this type of inquiry. The nine principles that he gave are (a) focusing on the "appearance of things" (p. 58); (b) being concerned for wholeness; (c) finding the essence of the appearance through intuition and reflection; (d) describing rather than analyzing; (e) having a personal interest; (f) asking questions that focus on integrating meaning, subject, and object; (g) understanding that "investigative intersubjective reality is part of the process" (p. 59); (h) using as primary evidence for investigation the researcher's intuition and reflection; and (i) very carefully and deliberately constructing the question being researched.

Moustakas (1994) investigated the methods and procedures that a phenomenological researcher uses to "… satisfy the requirements of an organized, disciplined, and systematic study" (p. 103). The first step he listed was to identify a topic and question "rooted in autobiographical meanings and values, as well as social meanings of significance" (p. 103). His second step was to conduct a thorough and comprehensive review of the professional literature in the area of the topic and the third to establish criteria to find the sample of "co-researchers" (p. 103) that will be used to study the topic. Fourth, Moustakas stated that the researcher must provide co-researchers with instructions about the purpose of the study and establish an agreement regarding confidentiality, informed consent, and a clear understanding of the procedures and meaning of involvement (p. 103). Moustakas's fifth step was to develop questions to guide the interview process and conduct in-depth interviews and follow-ups, if necessary, with the subjects (p. 103). Finally, he asserted that the researcher must organize and analyze the data found in the interview process and synthesize the data for their essence and meaning (p. 104).

This research study respects the Moustakas (1994) model as follows: First, I established questions through personal interest and my experience as a clinician-turned-executive director. Research in the area of mental health leadership, as well as needs identified by the Associate Director of The Ohio Council of Behavioral Health & Family Services Providers, suggest that the question of leadership development for mental health leaders is a relevant topic. Second, I established the criterion for co-researchers through working in conjunction with the Associate Director of The Ohio Council of Behavioral Health & Family Services Providers. Third, I determined that the research procedure will involve thoroughly introducing the topic to the participants. Fourth, I have crafted questions to draw out the phenomenon as it has been experienced. The questions used for the study are found in Appendix A. Finally, the data will be analyzed and the meaning of the information described.

Participants

Patton (2002) said the use of "purposeful sampling" (p. 272) in qualitative research is to carefully select research subjects who specifically represent the research question—this brings strength to qualitative inquiry. Investigating information-rich cases, he claimed, generates insights and deep understanding rather than empirical generalizations (p. 273). Patton (1990) put forth 16 sampling strategies designed to allow the researcher to select subjects salient to the research question (p. 182). Of those strategies, the one I have chosen to use for the present study is *intensity sampling* (Patton, 1990, p. 171). This technique is used when the researcher needs to find an information-rich sample that demonstrates the phenomenon being studied. The focus is on finding "excellent or rich examples of the phenomenon of interest but not unusual cases" (Patton, 1990, p. 171). Patton (1990) stated that this technique requires the researcher to determine the nature of variation in the phenomenon being studied so that the particular subjects can be selected.

In order to study the developmental process of CMHC executive directors, it was critical to investigate directors who have been in the field long enough to be able to have reflected on their experience of development from clinician to executive. It was also important to consider those who have the ability to articulate their experience. Because there are over 300 community behavioral health organizations in Ohio, I needed to narrow the selection of subjects to a sample group that can best reflect the developmental process. The Associate Director of The Ohio Council of Behavioral Health & Family Services Providers was used as a consultant in the role of gatekeeper to help select the sample. The reason for using the consultant in the selection process was that the consultant had a relationship at some level with all of the members of The Ohio Council of Behavioral Health & Family Services Providers and was be able to identify those who meet the above-mentioned criteria of having enough years in transition from clinician to director, as well as being able to self-reflect and verbalize the experience and discuss its impact on themselves. The gatekeeper identified a pool of 10 subjects. After we reviewed members of the group for their ability to provide an intense description of the phenomenon, we selected six for interview.

The following criteria were used to include the directors in the sample:

- They began their careers as clinicians.
- They have been directors at least four years.
- While they were in their role, the agency was successful in its mission, based on the following characteristics:
  - Based on agency outcome measures, most persons served indicate having improved because of the service of the agency.
  - Based on agency outcome measures, most persons served are satisfied with the treatment they received.
- Neither they nor the agency has any ethical violations of any kind.

After we identified the top six candidates, I approached them via phone to provide a brief description of the study, its purpose, goals, and procedures. Once the candidates agreed over the phone, I sent them the informed consent and interview questions via e-mail and scheduled face-to-face interviews with them at their respective agencies. At that interview, I presented the study in more detail and discussed their consent to participate and the privacy parameters. At that time, when the candidates agreed to be part of the study, I obtained their consent and signature to proceed with them in the study. I conducted the first interview at that time.

Research Questions

This study was guided by one primary question and three sub-questions. The primary question was, What is the developmental experience of CMHC directors who begin their careers as clinicians and become effective executive directors? The three sub-questions were as follows: (1) What do CMHC directors describe as the most helpful resources during this transitional process? (2) What are the most important lessons directors have learned through those resources? (3) What competencies did the directors consider to be most important for them to learn?

I collected data by conducting interviews on six subjects, each of whom participated in two interviews. The first interview focused on several questions (see Appendix A). centered on experiences, development, and resources. The second interview involved follow-up questions for areas that need clarification and that enabled the subjects to elaborate, without an interview guide, on how they describe their own development. Once the interviews were completed, the data were analyzed.

To guide the first interview, I posed 14 questions to each subject (see Appendix A). The questions were broken down into three categories. The first category consisted of questions that targeted the experiences directors have had as they have transitioned and worked as directors. The second category of questions focused on the developmental process each leader experienced. The final group of questions examined the resources the leaders identified as key to their experience. The interview questions were developed after I examined the type of information that would be needed to answer the primary and secondary research questions. Once I developed the questions to be used for the interviews, I conducted a pilot test on other leaders to increase their validity.

The interviews were digitally recorded on an audio device and were transcribed by a professional transcriptionist. Throughout the research, I also kept a journal that included observations I made during the interview, such as facial expressions, eye movements, or other nonverbal forms of communication. The journal was also a place to record my own thoughts and experiences throughout the research.

Analysis

To analyze the data in this study, I used a process of thematic analysis. I combined the models identified by Braun and Clarke (2006) and Creswell (2007), which complement and overlap each other. Whereas Braun and Clark (2006) emphasized the need for researchers to immerse themselves in the transcript to familiarize themselves with the data before identifying themes or codes (p. 87), Creswell (2007) emphasized the need for researchers to describe their personal experiences with the phenomenon. Creswell also highlighted the need for the researchers to describe, after identifying themes, what the participants experienced with the phenomenon and how the experience happened (p. 159). Both models emphasize the use of initial coding and theme development.

In following these two models, my first step was to completely familiarize myself with the transcripts of the interview data. I did this by reading the transcripts numerous times and taking time to meditate and reflect on the meaning of each participant's responses. After processing the interviews and their meaning, I generated initial codes by making notes on the transcripts and by highlighting with various colors that related to particular codes. In the next phase, I gathered the initial codes into potential themes that surfaced. After the initial themes were identified, I checked whether those themes worked with the scope of the entire data set and then used the themes to create a thematic map. Once the visual of the thematic map was created, I began to put the themes into the context of the story that they revealed and to generated definitions and names for each theme. At this point, I used verbatim examples to describe what the participants experienced with the phenomenon. Creswell (2007) described the technique of using the participants' descriptions of the phenomenon and including verbatim examples of their experience a "textural description" (p. 159). After the textural description, I completed a "structural description" (Creswell, 2007, p. 159) of how each subject's experience with the phenomenon transpired.

According to Creswell's (2007, p. 159) and Braun and Clarke's (2006, p. 96) outlines for phenomenological studies, once the data analysis has been completed the researcher then completes the written report, which will be found in the fourth chapter of this dissertation. The structure of this written report began by describing my own experience with the phenomenon. Once I discussed my experience, I used the themes found in the analysis of the interviews, along with the textural and structural descriptions of what each participant depicted, to portray the essence of the experience for the participant. This description tied back to the research question and the literature review to help frame the findings in the context of research in the field.

Trustworthiness

Merriam (2009) discussed the concepts of reliability and validity as they are applied in qualitative research. She suggested that, because the underlying assumptions of qualitative research are different from those of quantitative research, these concepts should be renamed to terms that more accurately reflect their use (Merriam, 2009, p. 211). In order to more accurately describe the trustworthiness of qualitative data, Lincoln and Guba (1985) used the terms *credibility, confirmability, dependability,* and *transferability* (p. 300). I have used these terms in this study.

Credibility

Lincoln and Guba (1985) used the term *credibility* to describe what would be known as "internal validity" in quantitative research (p. 300). The question asked to determine the credibility of the research is, "Are the findings credible given the data presented?" (Merriam, 2009, p. 213). To strengthen the credibility of my research, I used five methods suggested by Merriam (2009): triangulation (p. 215), member checks (p. 217), adequate engagement of the data (p. 219), "reflexivity" (p. 219), and peer review (p. 220). Following Merriam, I used triangulation by cross-checking my interpretations in three ways. First, I conducted two interviews with each subject. This dual process allowed me to clarify the statements they have made in the first interview. Second, I had three other professionals read my interpretations and evaluate and compare their interpretations with mine. For the professionals, I used doctorate-level mental health leaders who have done independent research work. They were given a hard copy of the draft of the analysis, as well as the transcripts, and I asked them to read the transcripts and the analysis. I then followed up with a phone call after two weeks and scheduled a meeting with them. In the meeting, each reviewer confirmed that my interpretation was an accurate representation of the interview data. Third, I compared my interpretations with other research in the field of health care leadership development and compared my explanations of the data to what others found as conclusions in their analyses.

After completing the cross triangulation, I enhanced the credibility of my data through member checking (Merriam, 2009). As I developed the analysis of the data, I checked with the participants to make sure that my descriptions were accurate. At the beginning of the second interview, I shared the major themes and codes that I identified and asked for feedback regarding their accuracy. After each second interview, I e-mailed the participants the textural and structural descriptions and ask for feedback. There were no discrepancies in their intended meaning and my interpretation

Using Merriam's (2009) third technique for enhancing credibility, I built in two interviews for each research participant rather than trying to accomplish all of the data gathering in one. By doing two interviews I enhanced the opportunities to more deeply explore the questions with each participant and gave him or her time to think over the answers and give additional information. In fact, the specific purpose of the second interview was to allow for clarification of meanings, as well as to allow the subjects to express their experiences without the use of questions to guide them.

My fourth technique to enhance credibility was reflexivity: The term *reflexivity* refers to my disclosing personal biases and how they have impacted the findings. I examined my own personal biases as they relate to the study. I accomplished this by recording my personal reflections and thoughts in a journal throughout the research project. This journal gave me insight into how I processed the information and reached conclusions regarding its meaning (Merriam, 2009, p. 219).

The fifth technique I used to enhance credibility was peer review. I asked three colleagues to review my work and assess the accuracy of my conclusions. The professionals I used were be doctorate-level mental health leaders who have done independent research work. They were given a hard copy draft of the analysis, as well as the transcripts. After a period of two to three weeks, during which they read the analysis, I met individually with each of them and received their feedback. Each of the peer reviewers concluded that my research analysis aligned with the transcripts and that my conclusions were accurate interpretations of the data.

Confirmability and Dependability

Merriam (2009) reported that confirmability in qualitative research correlates to the factor of reliability in quantitative research (p. 211) and suggested that, like reliability, confirmability means that if the study were replicated the results would be the same (p. 220). Merriam also clarified that qualitative research is not done so that "human behavior can be isolated. Rather researchers seek to describe and explain the world as those in the world experience it" (p. 220). Lincoln and Guba (1985) discussed the overlap of techniques to establish dependability and confirmability. Those authors mentioned the use of a "confirmability audit" (p. 318) that, if done properly, "can be used to determine dependability and confirmability simultaneously" (Lincoln & Guba, 1985, p. 318).

In this study, I used four techniques to augment both dependability and confirmability. Three of the four, already identified in the previous section, are triangulation, peer review, and reflexivity. The fourth technique used was a "confirmability audit" (Lincoln and Guba, 1985, p. 318). The confirmability audit included two components: the "audit trail" and the "audit process" (Lincoln and Guba, 1985, pp. 319–320). Lincoln and Guba (1985) discussed their concept of a confirmability audit as stemming from a dissertation done by Edward Halpern (1983) on the topic of auditing the confirmability of qualitative research. My audit trail consisted of the documents associated with my research and included the recorded interviews, transcripts, field notes, identified themes and data synthesis, field notes, and any other written or recorded material. The audit process followed the algorithm identified by Lincoln and Guba (1985, Appendix B). The first stage of the process was *preentry* (Lincoln & Guba, 1985, p. 321), which entailed a discussion with potential auditors and the selection of an auditor. The auditor completed a *determination of auditability* (p. 321) of my work based on the audit trail. Once it was determined that my project had adequate information to audit, we engaged in the third step, the *formal agreement* (p. 322). In this stage, the auditor and I established the time limit, goals, and other logistics for the audit. With an agreement established, the auditor began the process of the next step of the study, *determination of trustworthiness* (p. 323). In this phase, the auditor assessed whether or not the quality of the data, the processes, and the conclusions were valid and trustworthy. After concluding the assessment of the trustworthiness of the study, the auditor completed the final step, known as *closure* (p. 324). In this, the final stage, the auditor wrote his findings and included a "letter of attestation" (p. 325) regarding the dependability and confirmability of the research project.

Transferability

Merriam (2009) pointed out that transferability refers to external validity, or the ability for research to be applied to the general population. Generalizability in a statistical sense, she asserted, is not possible (p. 224). Lincoln and Guba (1985) stated that the burden of generalizability lies with the person trying to make the transfer, rather than with the original researcher (p. 298). They suggested that the best way to make the generalization is to "accumulate empirical evidence about the contextual similarity" (p. 298). Despite the stated challenges to transferability within qualitative research, Eisner (1991) pointed out that lessons are learned from life on a regular basis (p. 197). To improve the transferability of my research I used the technique suggested by Creswell (2009) of "rich, thick descriptions" (pp. 191–192). Prior to Creswell, Geertz (1973) had cited the importance of using thick descriptions in qualitative research, stating that the use of thick descriptions in ethnography "define the enterprise" (p. 6). Merriam (1998) suggested using descriptions that are rich and thick enough to allow readers to determine how well the study applies to the research they are doing. This richness allows the reader to make the transfer if appropriate. I used that level of detail as much as possible to add to the transferability of this research.

Lincoln and Guba (1985) suggested the use of a "reflexive journal" (p. 328) for the researcher to keep a record of his or her thoughts and experiences throughout the research process. During the course of my project, in order to provide another layer of accountability, I kept a journal of my thoughts, work, reflections, questions, decisions, issues, and interactions with the data, as well as any other pertinent information related to the process. The journal allowed me to track how I arrived at the interpretation of the interview information.

Ethics

Creswell (2009) cautioned researchers to anticipate the ethical issues that may arise during their studies (p. 87), and Merriam (2002) identified the areas of data collection, data dissemination, "researcher-participant relationship, ...privacy, and protection from harm" as areas in which ethical dilemmas could easily emerge (p. 29). Later Merriam (2009) stated that the reliability and validity of a study depend on the ethics of the investigator (p. 228).

In order to practice research in an ethical manner, I adhered to the American Counseling Association's (2005) *ACA Code of Ethics*. Participants were each given a copy of their interview transcripts, as well as the final interpretation of the meaning of their interview. They were given an opportunity to discuss with me any differences or discrepancies they had perceived. The feedback I received in all cases was that my interpretation accurately reflected the meaning that they, the participants, had intended.

Summary

Little, if any, research so far has described the developmental course of community mental health executive directors who began their career as clinicians. In Ohio, most of the leaders of the community mental health centers are nearing retirement. According to the Associate Director of The Ohio Council of Behavioral Health & Family Services Providers, there is a developing shortage of qualified leadership to step into place.

My study examined community mental health center executive directors who began their career as clinicians, and then described the developmental process that occurred as they progressed from clinician to director. This type of approach, exploring and telling the story of another's experience, stems from a social constructivist frame (Creswell, 2007; Guba & Lincoln, 1994). This paradigm was used so that the experience of development, as it was understood and perceived by the participants, could be accurately described. Because I sought in this study to discover the essence of the developmental experience of the individual leader, I used a phenomenological approach. The primary method of gathering data in this phenomenological study was interviewing.

The study explored the developmental course of six executive directors who lead community mental health centers in Ohio. Participants were selected with the help of the Associate Director of The Ohio Council of Behavioral Health & Family Services Providers. Directors who were effective in their jobs as well as able to describe their experiences were prioritized for selection. Through a set of predetermined questions, I gleaned their descriptions as to how they have developed as leaders. Once the information had been gathered, I extracted the essence of the data's meaning and described the phenomenon. The following chapter reports and explains the findings of the project.

CHAPTER IV

Results of Data Analysis

This research was an effort to present the developmental experience of executive directors of community mental health centers in Ohio who began their careers as clinicians. In order to do this, I engaged in a phenomenological study of six directors who work in various agencies throughout the state. I used adult development and adult learning as the theoretical frames. Demographically, the directors ranged in experience from 4 to 30 years of being in their role as executive director. The group interviewed was made up of two Caucasian females, three Caucasian males, and one African American male. The size of the agencies they were leading, based on budget, ranged from just over $1 million in annual revenue to $50 million in revenue. Their locations varied among rural, suburban, and urban settings.

The interviews were conducted over an eight-week period, and each director had an initial structured interview using 14 guiding questions (see Appendix A), along with a follow-up interview. The follow-up was used to clarify any questions I had after reviewing the first interview and to give the directors a chance to speak openly about their developmental experiences. During the second interview, I also asked each director which five pieces of advice he or she would give to new directors just beginning their careers.

Once the interviews were completed, I broke down the data analysis process in several stages. First, I read through each transcript to familiarize myself with them all individually. After I had familiarized myself with each transcript, I re-read them twice and began to record major themes that had surfaced. After identifying the themes found in the transcripts, I color-coded the transcripts by theme. Once the themes had been color-coded within each transcript, I then moved the coded data to an Excel spread sheet in which tabs were labeled by code, and segments of the transcripts were organized in each tab according to interviewee who made the statements that corresponded with each code. I then moved each of the coded pieces of data into two tabs that fit into the two emergent themes of "becoming a director" and "being a director." These tabs were organized by subthemes that arose from my analysis and placed in columns. That information was then woven into the Word document that became the rough draft of this chapter in a way that described the story of the phenomenon of the clinician-to-director development process. In order to protect the anonymity of the interviewees I have used alternating gender throughout this document.

I organized the data around the two major themes already mentioned, the first being "becoming a director." The information within this first major theme described what the interviewees experienced from the time they began their careers until they reached a point of feeling competent in their role. Within this major theme, seven subthemes made up the component of the overall experience of becoming a director: (a) an organic developmental process, (b) an early identification of administrative skills, (c) the attainment of an expanded worldview, (d) the impact of people along the way, (e) the growth of savvy, (f) an experience of growing pains, and (g) an identity shift.

Within the second major theme that emerged from the data, that of "being a director," six subthemes took shape: (a) the role of protector, (b) the reality of dealing with power, (c) the pressure experienced, (d) the importance of understanding and managing politics, (e) the effort of striving for authentic leadership, and (f) the importance of self-care. These six subthemes, combined with the seven subthemes for the experience of becoming a director, make up the phenomenon of the clinician-to-director process that the six directors experienced.

Becoming a Director

The theme of becoming a director developed from statements from the interviewee answers to the interview questions and from their descriptions of their experiences from the time they began their jobs as directors up through a point where they felt they had completed the process of developing into a director. The subthemes organize the data around the key elements of the interviewees' explanation of the developmental experience.

The seven subthemes include first, the directors describing their developmental experience as unique to them and impacted by many experiences they have had throughout their lives rather than either linear or cyclical. Second, the subthemes also entail the participating interviewees describing how early on in their careers they were recognized as having skills in supervising, managing, and leading that precipitated their being placed in positions of authority prior to becoming executives director. Third, the subthemes describe the directors' experience of growing their perspective of the business of community mental health from a simplistic understanding to a more complex picture that includes the financial, legal, and human resource aspects of the agency. Fourth, the subthemes describe how people and relationships have had a powerful impact on the development of the interviewees, as well as, fifth, how the experiences they have had, coupled with the demands of accomplishing the mission, forced them to grow more savvy in how they approached their work. The final two subthemes address the emotional challenges and growing pains the directors experienced as they were developing the necessary skills to be successful, and finally, how their professional identity has had to shift and grow into one that encompasses all of the roles an executive director fulfills.

Organic Developmental Process

As I explored whether the interviewees had experienced their development as linear or cyclical, what emerged was that the experience of development was not easily described using either term. When I asked the question, "So would you describe your experience, your development, your growth, as linear or cyclical?" the response from one director was "both." Another director said, "Certainly there's a linearity to it. I can see it. But all the cycles kind of play themselves through at every major developmental area, I think." Predominately, the responses indicated that the developmental experience was very individualized. One director who stated, "Well, I think as we sort of spoke at the beginning, it's been a convoluted path to my current position.... So no, it has not been linear in any way," went on to clarify how his development was impacted by the people with whom he had had opportunities to interact:

> Yeah, every individual is different, so you see somebody, or I would see somebody, who pays attention to detail, and I'd see the benefits of that ... take something away from that, ... see somebody who is real creative and take something away from that. So I think every person takes something, at least every person that I admire or I think is accomplished.... I'll take something away from that direction.

Another director discussed that growth as resembling child and adult development:

> I would say it's a lot like the developmental stages that you have when you are growing up. They may not be the same, but I think that as a leader there's probably stages you go through. And I would characterize it ... it's kind of like I've gone through my infancy now, and I feel like I'm probably somewhere in my adolescence as far as where I'm grown up. I'm not quite to the adult level yet.

For the directors interviewed, the developmental process encompassed many aspects of their lives, not only their work experiences. One put it this way:

> And then you may need to go back a little further, and then you may come full circle, and then that may come up again in a different situation. Linear in that I think that every learning that I have about myself and about the organization lends itself to an enhanced view—which I think of as linear—an enhanced view of who I am as a person, as a leader, and who we are as an agency. And so I'm constantly adding to that. Linear in that when I think about strategic planning, I just think about that as being linear ... that I am setting goals, I am setting timelines. And

some of those goals and timelines I'm setting for myself, and I need to make changes as a leader so that I can reach those.... I mean, like, for example, I remember something that helps me now. I remember something now that my grandfather always used to say to me that helps me now with what I did. And it's helped me throughout my entire professional career ... and with regard to risk-taking and whatnot.

Another director, in summing up how various experiences had impacted him and whether or not he saw the development as linear or cyclical, stated, "I think each experience made me stronger, made me a better leader ... even though going through it was certainly not pleasant. But the lessons that I learned are still, I mean, very much alive." This organic process, which each director was able to describe, was often supported by a number of leadership opportunities for the directors as their careers developed. These opportunities were a component that all of the directors discussed. For each one, people had identified, early on in their career, that they had skills in leadership.

Early Identification of Leadership Skills

All of the directors I interviewed stated that they began their training for becoming an executive director early in their career. Their skills in leadership were identified early on by supervisors or peers and they were chosen to serve in various leadership and administrative roles. For example one research participant, over the course of her career, had supervised case management teams, counselors, and even the billing department prior to becoming the executive director. Another was asked to become a clinical director and yet another asked to be the assistant director, all before stepping into the role of executive director. For some, these early leadership experiences made the transition to executive director less of a jump. For others, the role of executive director was so different from their other experiences that it was a very big adjustment.

Five out of six of the directors I interviewed were able to describe an experience of leadership aptitude early on in their careers as clinicians. As one director put it, "I thought I was good at it. People thought I was good at it." Another director felt that although he took on leadership roles he continued to view himself as fulfilling an essential role on the team and that he was simply a member of the team. He stated that although he had had many opportunities to learn administration, those roles were not different from the staff roles he was supervising, "still very much sharing physical space with those that were out on the front lines; and really acting in the role of guide and just as a part of the team that has a different level of skill sets."

The evolution from being a clinician whose focus was singularly on client care to being a leader who was responsible for the entire organization occurred for the directors as they had opportunities to take on new roles. Sometimes they were noticed by people working at other agencies in their community who had observed their leadership skills. One director was approached by another organization's executive director: "I don't have a clinical director, are you interested?" When the opportunity presented itself, she reported that she , "…jumped at the opportunity to work with bigger pictures." She was then approached by another agency, "and the clinical director approached me and said that their executive director was leaving. And she said that ... you know ... I really think you should apply for that job." Another director described being identified early on as a good administrator, "then took on the role of client rights specialist. And so I wore a number of different hats.… I continued to grow as the agency grew, and as I continued to [grow], my job title changed." A similar experience is described as, "I became an administrator, and so I supervised people doing clinical service. But I started our first programs in the community for people who are homeless. I supervised all of those. And then I transitioned from that to being the organization's associate executive director."

The administrative opportunities for each of these directors along the way, such as being a manager or supervisor, helped prepare them for the eventual evolution into an executive director in which they were responsible for the entire organization instead a portion of it. Each step allowed the directors to learn key pieces of the job. One director described it as follows:

> As the executive director I had to understand how to read an audit, and I had to understand general accounting procedures. I had to understand investments.… And what would be another example? When I was incorporating new companies, making new companies, I had to learn about intellectual property.… I had to learn about labor law. So I couldn't have managed that company without understanding about legal [issues] and law.

These experiences allowed some of the directors to feel as though they were prepared for the next step of becoming an executive director. One example of this is, "So it wasn't the jump for me. It wasn't directly from clinician to executive director. There had been quite a number of years that I had not done the actual clinical work myself." Another said, "So by the time I did full-time administration, I had a range of other experiences that are endemic to being an executive director."

One of the interviewees summed up how personal experience in various administrative roles evolved and put her in what she felt was the right place for her:

> If you kind of flow where it takes you.… That sounds sort of ... I think, it's half of what you bring to the world and half of what the world brings to you. So sometimes it's a nice fit. And if you go with that fit between your readiness and what the world presents, you don't fight it. It takes you somewhere, and that's where it took me. And it just seems like it was never a big discrete change; it just evolved.

This early identification of administrative skills and the experience that followed clearly helped the directors evolve into the executive director role. Once they had reached the position of executive director, however, four out of the six interviewees indicated that they had to learn to navigate in a much larger world than ever before; they had to develop an expanded worldview.

Expanded Worldview

As the directors discussed their transformation from clinician to director, two thirds of them described how their view of what encompassed the operations of a CMHC vastly expanded. They were able to describe how, as clinicians, their focus was on the patients they served and all of the tasks involved in accomplishing the day-to-counseling sessions and how, once they were administrating, the responsibilities around finance and leadership quickly took them into another dimension.

One director described that particular transformation this way:

I think what I didn't realize was [that] as a clinician your view of the agency is so small, and [there are] many other things that go on that you have no idea about. It's like you go from being, like, a little sheltered—like, all I have to worry about is the small set of paperwork and rules—to this huge world that you didn't know even existed as far as accreditations and re-certifications, finances, budgeting ... all the things that your education, as far as counselor, didn't cover.

In an effort to put this experience in the context of development, another director said,

Well, I think when people are trained to be clinicians, they don't get a good understanding of the broader context, the broader, non-clinical contexts: what it takes to actually support oneself, to [work] in an agency. As a clinician, you ... [only see] a much more narrow view of things.

Yet another perspective on development was

to jump from there [being a clinician] to dealing with funding agencies and all the extremes of money and how that's done. And I think as a clinician you don't at all realize what it takes to run an organization ... and you're kind of shielded from all the financial pieces that, as long as things are running, you're ... you know, units of service, all those things you have to produce.

In describing the larger world of a director versus the world of a clinician, one director stated,

[At] 2:00 you're dealing with the accounting firm, 3:00 you're dealing with the law firm, and 5:00 you're dealing with a donor. And before that you were dealing with a clinician. So you're dealing with a wider variety of people, and they all have their own agendas. Many of [them] are accomplished, if not more accomplished than you. You're dealing with politicians.

The experience of learning this bigger world is overwhelming, as revealed by one director describing the first few months as director: "Back then, you know, how naive ... how naively you walk into things. You're pulled in so many directions. And there are so many things that you need to learn so rapidly." In further describing the stressful period of seeing the bigger picture, this director went on to say, "But it was a much bigger jump for me to make that leap at that point and to understand funding streams and how it is that the organizations dissolved. And I also got my first view of politics at that point. In comparing the views, one director summarized that the counselor's role is much simpler, "because the counseling piece is pretty small when you figure in finances, strategic planning, accreditation, state regs, [and] building maintenance."

When asked what would help a new director be better able to integrate this new view, one director said,

Continuing education in just about anything would be helpful: finance, strategic planning, fundraising. There's a whole ... a great amount of information out there about those other things. And realizing our shortcomings, what we didn't really have. Our education isn't based in these business kinds of things, and I think for any new director, get as much information as you can absorb about those other things so that you can understand the whole picture a little bit better.

Another director discussed the importance of relying on the other surrounding professionals in leadership:

So I've learned more about it than I ever wanted to know, but I still don't know what I think I should know as a person in this position.... But that's why I'm glad that I have good people who I know that I can trust. Because they can say ... even if I don't understand, they go, "Yeah, well, I'll explain it to you later, but it's got to go in today to the board, so just sign it."

This larger worldview was a major adjustment for the interviewees, and one of the ways in which they were able to learn to manage it was with the help of other professionals or people in their lives. All interviewees, in fact, highlighted the impact of people's input on their growth over the course of time during which they became directors.

The Impact of People

When I asked the directors what resources had helped them grow, all of them commented on people who had helped them develop as they moved along in their journey from clinician to director. Asked what resources helped the most, one director simply put it like this: "Mostly people. Good people can teach you a lot about yourself.... You know, I would give most of the credit to those people." Three of those interviewed talked about members of their board of directors as being key. One stated, "And my executive committee has been just essential in the growth process in helping me move on." Another said, "It was the voice of several of our board members who took me under their wing.... They recognized what I was up against."

When mentioning people as a key resource in their development, others talked about the staff they worked with. One said, "I've had some wonderful supervisors in the past. I've had some wonderful colleagues ... some wonderful people I work with here. I'm pleasantly surprised everyday what people do for good [causes]." Another declared,

> Those around me. This group. The directors. Who I had, you know, been a part of at one point. They were and are my biggest cheerleaders. And they ... at points where I, especially in those early ... that first year ... had doubts—they had none.

One of those interviewed spent time talking about a previous supervisor who had a lasting impact on the style of leadership the interviewee adapted. This interviewee stated, "He was a Ph.D. at the time. I was in a terminal master's in clinical psych.... So I was working as a psych assistant then. And I learned as much as I could from him." Another director discussed how college academic advisors had helped shape the leadership style he adopted:

> Actually I've always been one of those people who thinks that you can learn something from anybody. I can learn ... allow myself to even learn from little kids even.... And I think my academic advisors that I chose and my internship advisors that I chose, you know, I got to be ... I chose them because of their reputations and what I had known about the work that they had done with other people and the respect that others had for them. So that's kind of how and why I chose them. And that also helped me.... I saw them doing the same things with me and caring and teaching and coaching and supporting me in the same way. And I was able to develop friendships with all of them, and that helped. And I developed a lot of those.

Some of the directors discussed how they learned "what not to do" from some of the leaders they either experienced or observed. One illustrated learning from a negative leadership encounter by describing the aftermath of the negative leader's tenure: "[The staff and board] had in many ways been disempowered by our past leader." Another director described a different situation with a previous leader:

> [The leader] was not the same person no matter who [he was] with. And certainly a much different person with the board than ... with the staff than ... with [the] executive team. And I didn't like that.... I just didn't like that.... Some of [his] anger issues just got in the way.

Whether because they were supportive, directive, a good example or a bad one, it seems the consensus was that people were the greatest resource for growth. One director summarized it best, saying, "The people I work with, you know, my employees, my board. I think they were key." Learning from people thus was an important aspect of the becoming-a-director process.

Becoming Savvy

Along with learning from people, the directors also had to learn more savvy ways of dealing with people. Growing savvy was a subtheme described by five out of the six interviewees. Five of the directors mentioned that over the course of their development they learned to be savvy in dealing with others, particularly in the political realm. One director put it this way when asked about some of the ways he had changed: "I think learning how to deal with a wide variety of other people, a wider variety of other people in a situation that's not ... [that] I don't have control over because I'm not the therapist." This director was explaining how as a therapist one has a greater amount of control over the work one does versus the variety of types of relationships one must successfully manage as a director.

Another director described the early part of this learning process by saying, "but there were lots of other powers at work at that point that I didn't really understand.... But it was interesting to watch that process ... the business relationships with the boards.... I began to understand a little more of the business side." The interviewee went on to describe learning to work with local politics. "This county ... I had to learn ... it's the first time I really had to cultivate relationships with sister agencies in a different way and become part of a whole system. Because we were in a fishbowl." This same director further explained how some of those relationships were managed: "There were a lot of things to learn there. The biggest thing was working with board members and understanding how that went. And in my naiveté, I think I just did the right thing. I just charged right in." From these experiences this director learned that being shrewd was an important tactic in managing relationships:

I learned a couple things right off the bat. One is that you can't always be totally transparent initially, because lots of times if you're dealing with macro issues, you've got a lot of things you need to put together and understand first, and gather as much information from everybody as you can ... but knowing that it influences everybody's job, they can't help you with decisions ultimately.

Another director shared learning this cautious approach as a part of development,

Well, I think that early on while I played more from my gut, I probably acted ... I was probably a little bit more rigid, more structured. So now that I'm more of a mix, I actually feel people would probably say I'm a little bit more of a cowboy on the outside, [but] ... I suppose I'm a bit more cautious.

Yet another director described the lessons of becoming savvy that came along with personal experiences:

You know, the amount of growth it has taken me to learn the systems and get my toes stepped on numerous times and go back at it the next day and put myself in a room full of people that I don't know and try to get along and talk to them and not say something stupid.

Another example from the interviewees included facing challenges with those they had to be able to work with in the community, "the experience of butting heads with [a local political leader] and to be able to say to them, 'I don't agree.' And then to be able to step away and to say, 'You know what, perhaps that conversation should have gone a different way.'"

Being savvy with others (being able to navigate these complex political relationships), whether with the staff, the board, other agencies, or local, state, or federal political entities, was a skill all considered important. On the other end of this learning curve, all of the directors were able to describe how they use political skill to their agency's advantage. All of them had to learn that in the end it is about managing relationships with people. One director, in particular, summed it up: "You know, so as I've gotten older, it hasn't mattered whether it's a U.S. senator or a presidential candidate or ... I don't know ... a city council member. People are people."

These five subthemes — organic developmental process, early identification of administrative skills, expanded worldview, impact of people, and growing savvy — all help describe the process of becoming a director. What underlies all of them, however, is the stress of learning new skills. All of the directors described such growing pains.

Growing Pains

All six of the directors interviewed described some level of stress or anxiety that allowed them to reach a point of competence as a director. They mentioned a variety of circumstances or experiences that were painful but yet helpful in their progress to understanding how to do the job. For instance, one director said, "And the other thing that forced me to grow was we had a horrible financial year ... for a bunch of reasons." That person went on to describe specifically how difficult financial decisions were a part of the growth process,

> And I've had to make some big decisions, some budget cuts that I had to do unilaterally. Even most of my executive committee team agreed, and the board was kind of in place with it. But I learned that I had to do that. And I believe that, as a consequence of that, I could do that and people accepted that. They weren't happy with some of the things we had to do because it affected us all.

The process of making those budget cuts then led to having to overcome some of this director's personality traits that made such choices more difficult:

> What else I learned about myself was that I have a tendency to be very empathetic to anybody's pain all the time. And I've learned that [there are] certain times that I can still feel the empathy, but I still need to make a decision that's difficult to make.

Another director discussed having to work through being bothered by others talking about him behind his back and being mischaracterized by others:

> I guess it used to bother me a little more that people might be saying things about me that weren't necessarily true. Or characterizing me in ways that weren't necessarily accurate. But over time I learned that, one, there's nothing I can do about it. People are going to talk.

Along with managing financial challenges and being the target of misinformation, another director discussed how the job pushes her beyond her comfort zone by necessitating decisions without a lengthy time to analyze and plan,

> [The job is] pushing me into places where I'm not comfortable. It's unfamiliar territory. I cannot do my six months of research to get comfortable with it. There may not be any research out there to look at. This may be completely ... I'm out here winging it altogether, and I'm not really a good winger.

This same director discussed how failing and risk-taking actually helped with learning and contrasted failure to risk-taking as a learning tool. "I would say failure has probably [taught me] more [about both] failure and risk. My personal philosophy is if you ... if you aren't failing, then you aren't trying very hard." Describing the process of learning to use risk as a tool this director said,

> I think risk is a really important piece of the job. And I think it's ... I think in this climate, if we're going to carve out our niches, some of it [is] you have to go into it with some realistic expectations that every risk that you take is not going to pay off.... But if you're not doing the risk, you're not going to make it because you need to [keep] carving out these niches.

The leaders also were able to describe how they made sense of the growing process. For some it was a gradual, slow process; others felt they had to ramp up quickly. One stated, "There was [not one] moment in time where, you know, I suddenly had self-realization. It was more gradual." Another said,

> I don't think that I've learned to do that [much] better or differently as a result of being a director necessarily. I think a lot of it comes through experience. Like many things in life, it's experience. The more you do something and the more successes you have with it, the more you learn about it and the better you get with it. So I don't think it's as much a function of the position as the opportunity and the experience.

A third director described it a bit differently: "And learning as much as you could as rapidly as you can and realizing that no one's got the truth, the light, and the way. And that I certainly don't, much of the time."

Whether they viewed it as a slow or fast process, one director summed up the reality quite well:

> A true leader, and I believe in that ... I think it has to be a constant process. And it will always be something new to learn, something more to develop ... something to do with change as we move along. And some of that is external forces acted on, but some of it needs to be internal, as well.

As the directors were able to describe a stressful growing process, many of them also were able to describe how their leadership skills have been impacted on the other side: "I'm learning to be more decisive and less wishy-washy. I definitely am more decisive. I want to make sure that I'm making a good choice; I'm not being impulsive about it, but making decisions more quickly," stated one interviewee. Another said, "I'm a little more cautious, just using numbers and the law department.... I use numbers more." A third director described himself by saying, "I'm more creative than what I [thought I was originally]. But that creativity ... also uses a blend of better planning than I did before.... And I learned pretty quickly that I really had to think things through." A fourth director was able to put her transformation and growth process into these words:

I am a more competent leader now, and that has more to do with my own personal growth around accepting the title. [All] around, I am not embracing the title, but I am accepting it and I am wearing mistakes, which is, I think, for the first six months of wearing this hat—well, I don't sleep anyway, but my sleep was just ... was just full of symbols of failure. I am now wearing ... I mean, who the hell am I to be carrying, at that point it was a $15 million agency; we're at $20 [million] now. What the hell? In whose world could this be happening? Because I am just me.

This person went on,

It's a story of transcendence, it's a story of transformation. And it's not just my story, it's the organization's story. And it's the story of how we as leaders have begun to experience our own strength in leading, have been able to reach out in even more important ways to the community, to those whose lives are shattered. That we have the ability to offer a hand is only because we are getting in touch with our own [best self].

The growth process described by the directors had a beginning and also a point at which they began to see themselves as directors rather than directors-in-training. For this to happen, the directors had to go through a final process of identity change, from becoming to being. Each one, in some way, discussed that identity shift.

Identity Shift

All of the directors discussed, in varying ways, undergoing an identity shift after experiencing the growing pains of the clinician-to-director transition. They began their work as directors seeing themselves in one way and, through the forge of experiences, they arrived at a new level of understanding who they are. For some, it was a dramatic transformation of their identity; for others it was as subtle as realizing how their personality affected others and altering it to a degree. For instance one director stated,

The first year that I was in this position I had a very difficult time introducing myself as, "I'm [name], the executive director." And part of that was my own internal sense of who I was and, you know, going back through ... there's all sorts of stuff going back to my childhood. And it's all about self-worth. And then I practiced. I actually practiced in the car, "Say your name. Say your name. You know, say your name, say your title. Practice that. What does that feel like?" That was a difficult hurdle to get over ... to be able to, through experiences and accepting the CEO construct ... to chisel away at that [reticence] till it was nothing but a pile of rubble. That was pretty cool. It would never have happened if I hadn't taken this job. I would still be walking around going, "He was right" [speaking of a co-worker who had promoted a negative self-image for this director].

Another director who also described a remarkable shift stated,

I think I have "counselor" somehow tattooed on my forehead.... And that's our spirit; to be a good clinician you have to.... I kind of thought I would be clinical director forever.... So the thread that weaves the tapestry of my life from clinician on through was the naive [new executive director] ... I think, kind of ... I think basically good natured and trying to be cooperative, as helpful as you can be.... [Now] I'm not as tolerant of the bullshit as I used to be.

One director discussed the transformation in more detail,

I think—yeah, I think the counselor in us wants to believe people are going to get better. Even the employees, they're going to get better.... Yeah, I think this job has changed me probably pretty drastically as a person. I am ... I still hold on to some of my idealistic features. But I'm much more realistic as a person now.... I mean, I have such a broader view of the world. That, yeah, it's really changed kind of the way I think about things, the way I process information, the way I interact with people. I mean, it's definitely impacted me.

This same director used human development terms to express how he saw his growth.

And I say, so that's doubly transformed me as a person. I think that—I know that this is big, but I think it's made me more mature.... I'm still an adolescent, still got a lot to learn. I still make a fair amount of mistakes.... And I think growing as a leader is the exact same way. You start out as a naive little baby, and you kind of [need to] grow up, and ... you do: You stick your finger in the light socket and, yeah, that hurt. I probably shouldn't do that anymore.

Another director described feeling like a peer to subordinate staff but having to accept being understood by the staff as the leader and needing to fill that role for them:

But sometimes that's hard for me to reconcile, because I guess I try at every opportunity possible to break down some of those hierarchical kinds of things.... I guess that would be it ... is just by how I want to view myself or what I think I am or how I think I fit into the equation or the organizations or society. Other people are going to continue to separate me out from that and look at me differently just by the nature of the title of the position that I'm in.

That leader discussed wrestling with staff over that identity as leader, very much wanting to be defined as just one of the team, although the staff could not allow it. This director had to take on the identity of the leader:

I know that there's that ... and staff have told me ... that there's that theme. But you are a boss, and no matter how much you tell us we can disagree or that we don't have to do it this way, there's still something ... you know, the subconscious or preconscious inside of us that's going to say, no, that's what he's saying, so that's what I've got to do.

The data from the interviews that were just presented described the phenomenon of "*becoming* a director." This phenomenon was comprised of seven subthemes including the directors discussing their development as being an organic process rather than one that could be labeled linear or cyclical. They discussed being noticed early on in their careers as having administrative and leadership skills. Once in the job they found that when they viewed the work of community mental health as having much more complexity it required them to expand their view of what it takes to accomplish the mission. They also described how they were impacted by various relationships along the way, how the complexities of the work or of leading required them to become more savvy. Finally, they described the experience of pain and stress they incurred during this time of becoming a director, which in the end led them to having a new and professional identity that encompassed the job of leading the organization. Although this description comprised a major portion of the information that came through in the interviews, the other major theme was "*being* a director." On this latter theme, which will be discussed in the following section, the interviewees described what it meant to function as, be recognized as, and take on the role of the top leader in a community mental health center.

Being a Director

The focus of this study was on exploring and describing the developmental process of executive directors of community mental health centers who began their careers as clinicians. The previous section presented information about how the subjects reported that experience for themselves. During the course of the interviews, however, another theme emerged as the directors described what it was like to be a director once they had gone through that initial developmental experience. The experience of *being a director* that came forward is made up of six subthemes. Within the subthemes the participants described being a director as encompassing the role of protector of the mission of the agency, the staff, and the business aspects of the agency. Another subtheme revolved around dealing with the power inherent in the job. The participants described feeling the weight of their power, the reality of having the final say, the consequences of power, and at times the perceived absence of power. Those interviewed also emphasized the pressure of the job by discussing where the pressures came from, describing the pressure and what it felt like. The directors discussed how important political skills were to the job for managing both external and internal political forces. Being self-aware, genuine, and reflectively seeking feedback emerged as a subtheme of the directors as they pursued an *authentic leadership* framework (Avolio & Gardner, 2005; Gardner et al., 2005; Luthans & Avolio, 2003; Walumbwa et al., 2008) to characterize their style. The final subtheme centered on the participants explaining the importance of self-care in order to be able to do the job successfully over the long haul.

The Role of Protector

The concept of being the protector of the agency manifested itself in all of the interviews. The directors described it in various ways and forms. The three ways that the directors visualized their role as protector manifested in three subthemes: protecting the mission, protecting the staff, and protecting the business.

Protecting the mission. The directors I interviewed feel a deep sense of obligation to focus on preserving and protecting the mission of the agency they work for. Sometimes this role of protector makes them unpopular with staff. One director summed up that responsibility in this way:

> So one of the big transitions was understanding that there were times that I got to make a decision for the good of all the people we serve, first, [and] second, for the agency to move that forward. And thirdly, [those decisions] aren't going to be wildly popular with everybody a lot of the time.

Another director rather humorously noted, "But sometimes the decisions that I have to make for the good of the agency ... I end up with a lot.... I always say it's a good day if no one cries."

There are various aspects of acting as agency protector. Within the context of the interviews, often this involved the task of eliminating staff who either harmed the people or the organizations served or who overall were not a good fit for the agency. One director stated powerfully the importance of

> being clear about the values that you hold for the organization, as well as for the individuals who are working within the organization. And [being] clear about repercussions if expectations aren't met, and not in a punitive way, but in a clarifying way.... I think of it as protecting the agency. Because if you have too many individuals that are not carrying the mission, and they are interspersed with those that are, it pulls the others down.... And so that was really powerful for me. This recognizing that, you know what, [in] nurturing an organization and those that are part of the organization, also there has to be some sense of protecting the ethics, the values, and what it is we define that is part of who we are.

The director went on to further define this issue of protecting the agency:

> I was not going to tolerate someone who strayed too far outside of what we had identified as being acceptable. Especially in terms of behaviors or attitudes towards, again, our clients, those that we served.... And I have to say, and I say it with some sense of pride, that probably within the first year, year and a half, we terminated more people than we had the five years prior. Because there were individuals that simply weren't doing their jobs ... even though they were provided redirection. And my thing is we give the people the opportunity to succeed, we provide clarification around what it is we expect to see. You get one or two chances every step of way, and then if you don't choose to embrace that, then we have to talk about that this is no longer a match.

Another director, in agreement with the idea of protecting the persons they served by making sure the staff was ethical and committed to the mission, stated,

> And when you have somebody that's going to be involved in some sort of abuse, neglect, or exploitation—and those are generally the primary reasons why we've had to fire staff who work with our patients—then I have no tolerance ... no patience with, yeah, you got in this business for the wrong reason, and you don't need to be in it.

One of the directors looked at the issue of protecting persons served from unethical staff as

> [The message I give staff is] you are here to do a job, and you are here to do a job in a specific way, however that's defined. And if we give you enough opportuni-

ties to succeed and [if] you choose not to take those, then you don't—you do not deserve, if you will—to be here.

One director summed up this aspect of protecting the agency as follows: "And I wish I didn't have to fire as many people as we do. But [then] there's some of these things that you just can't abide by." Another director viewed the concept of his role as protector of the mission in relation to the organization's impact on the community, particularly as he represented a rather large organization that had a significant financial impact on the region in which it was located. This director discussed how he felt the need, as director, to protect not only the agency but the impact the agency had on the community as it carried out its mission. He framed it as follows:

> Yeah, I have a greater sensitivity to the community at large.... So it's just because of the size [that the agency] impacts a lot more people.... You have a greater responsibility for greater and greater community. You see yourself as part of ... more of mankind or more of community.... So if you screw up here, it affects jobs in Ohio.

Protecting the staff. Along with the role of protecting the agency by protecting its mission, the directors also identified the role of protector by protecting the staff. The concern was expressed at two different levels. One of the directors, speaking out of the weight she felt for providing financial stability for her staff, stated, "I feel a greater responsibility for people's mortgages." The other director who discussed this particular notion of being the protector discussed the importance of making sure that staff, who very often were victims of vicarious trauma through the patients they serve, were able to receive the support they, in turn, needed in order to carry on: "It's my responsibility," he said, "to make sure that I've built in opportunities for them to experience their own strength and their own healing."

Protecting the business. The third nuance to the role of protecting identified by the directors is in relation to how they protect the business aspects of the organization. All of the directors articulated that focusing on the business was a key aspect of their role as executive director and as protector of the organization so that it could accomplish its mission. One director explained, "... because you go from being concerned about the peer group to [where] your main concern has to be the survival of the corporation. It doesn't do the staff or the clients any good if you're not around anymore." Another director stated, "And it can't be about just that individual [staff] person's feelings or needs. It has to be about how the agency is run. It has to be about client care, making sure we're doing good client care."

In discussing this aspect of their role, two of the directors described hiring the right staff and placing staff in their correct roles as key to protecting the organization. One stated,

> There have been things that I have never let go of ... things I've never delegated. One is hiring, the other is firing. Nobody gets hired or fired in this place unless I say so. And that's a protection for employees as well as supervisors.

The other said, "I'm doing it for the right reasons. And it's not about me getting my needs fulfilled. It's really about the agency and doing that ... and making sure the right people are in the right jobs doing the right thing."

In summing up how their independent roles as protectors of the agency's mission, clients, and staff are all an integrated part of the position of director, one director stated, "This is about carrying the heart and the soul as well as the responsibility of serving individuals and taking care of our staff ... being kind of the director of the orchestra." One more example is,

> When I am speaking with a voice of the CEO—and it's imperative that I do, because I can do a lot of damage if I don't—what I say carries a lot of weight because of my title.

In describing the need to be viewed by staff as the protector of the agency, a director stated,

> It's always part of a questioning and a recognizing that it may not be how I see myself, but I need to be aware how others view me. And I need to be aware that I—and I've always kind of carried this—that I am a role model.

Finally, one director defined the protector role as "for you to understand that ultimately you're accountable to the organization." Another put it more simply: "I'm responsible for everything that happens here."

The role of protector thus inherently carries power within it: Directors are given power to release or fire employees they feel are not performing in the best interest of the organization, to hire staff they believe will best help with achieving the agency's mission, to put policies and procedures into place that allow the organization to run effectively, and to make decisions that allow the agency to move forward both when planning for the long term and when dealing with times of crisis. Most of the directors interviewed considered the reality of power a significant component of their job.

The Impact of Power

The aspect of being a director and fulfilling the role of protecting the agency was one with which all of the directors identified. This role places on the director the responsibility of protecting the mission, the persons served, the staff, and the business. Because of these three facets it is also a powerful function. Five of the six directors discussed the aspect of power associated with being an executive director. They discussed power in four ways. The first was related to the idea of carrying the power and the weight of the power being carried. The second was related to organizational decision making and having the final say in an organizational setting. The third way these directors discussed power was in relation to the consequences their power has in the life of the organization, employees, and persons served. Finally, some mentioned that they actually feel powerless, despite having great authority. The four aspects of power were described in the following way by the interviewees:

The weight of power. The directors all indicated at some level the sense of the power that resides within the position they hold in the agency. One director, in particular, described feeling the weight the power of the position holds and how it impacted him, "that there is this, you know, this heavy power that I carry." That director went on to describe his struggle with accepting the power of the position. His struggle resided in the fact that he had seen power in a position such as that of executive director wielded in a way that primarily used the tools of manipulation and intimidation to manage staff and other leaders:

> I think some of my greatest struggles around becoming a CEO had to do with power, had to do with changing the way power looked.... You know, the accepting of power, being worthy of having power.... Usually when I think of power, it's with dark letters.... Power was something that was very painful, especially for the executive leadership team.

This particular director was able to have a positive experience in his role, and it became transformative in his view of power: "Power now is something that is light. It's transformative. It's translucent. It's something that helps one grow." Discussing how experience with power had changed his view, he said,

> You know, I come back to the word *power*—that I am closer to being able to embrace power if I give it a different definition ... or because I am giving it a different definition. And because the culture has shifted. Because we have, for the most part, healed as an organization [from an experience with a different administrator].

70

Having the final say. The directors who spoke about power conceived it at times as a very heavy aspect of their role. One key way in which they found it heavy is that they are ultimately responsible for everything that goes on in their organization. In essence, the buck *does* stop with them.

In regard to the idea that "the buck stops here," one director added, "and I have to draw that bottom line alone many times." Another director discussed how she felt the aspect of power related to decision making impacted staff. She also described how, although she likes to be inclusive in decision making, often she needs to make choices based on information she alone possesses: "[Then] I'm going to have to make a unilateral decision." Speaking of how she hoped the staff received the decision-making process, she said,

> And I hope that you get to know me well enough to know that if I have to do that ... it's the only way I could have done it given all the givens, and that ... and I was balanced and fair in the process.

In the end, however, this director stated, "When it comes down to it you just have to do it."

Consequences. Along with the finality of responsibility for decision making within their organizations, the directors had a keen sense of the consequences of the power inherent within their jobs, and they discussed how they experienced the end results of their power and decision making. For example, one said, "Your decisions don't just affect the bottom line, you know, but people die if your folks make the wrong decision; and people prosper and recover if you do the right thing."

All of the directors discussed how the consequences of their power could make the organization either better or worse. Said one,

> I have the ability to reach out to others and to get input and so I can base decisions on that. And the lesson that I have learned is that that is a pretty powerful thing to do as a CEO.... I have the power to be able to say, "By God, this is what we need to do." And then to make sure it happens.

Or, on the hard side of this decision-making power, as one director put it, "I may have to fire you at some point."

The perceived absence of power. In both indirect and direct ways at least three of the directors discussed their sense of powerlessness in relation to their positions. One director in particular addressed it directly: "The feedback I've gotten, you know, it's kind of a powerful thing. And believe me, when I'm in the role I don't feel that powerful.... I don't." He went on to describe how his powerlessness manifests itself day to day in his role,

> and one of the things that I thought about was just because you're the boss that doesn't mean people do what you say to do. They'll do a version of it. They'll say they do, [but] they don't do it at all. And that's what's difficult to reconcile ... that just because you're boss—I think I said this to you—you're just not all that powerful.

As another example, he stated, "Just because I'm the boss doesn't make them believe me."

The conclusion that this director came to was that, in relation to the power of the position and its impact on staff accomplishing the mission, "the only real way to get people to do what you want is to get them to buy into you." Thus along with this sense of power and all of its facets, and along with the role of protector, comes an incredible amount of pressure.

Pressure

All of the directors spoke in one way or another about the amount of pressure they feel they have in this job. For some, as mentioned before, it is related to the weight of the responsibility they feel to their mission, staff, or community. The pressure that the directors feel emerged as another major component of the role of being a director. The pressure that the interviewees described fell into three groupings. The first was simply an identification of the pressure they felt regarding different aspects of their job, the second was a description of the pressure that came from a feeling of loneliness related to being in the job, and the third was a series of comments describing what the pressure from the job felt like.

Identifying the pressure. The directors mentioned many aspects of their job that caused them to feel pressure, including making decisions that were going to have a great impact on their organizations and human resources decisions, such as firing someone or laying off staff. A director described it this way: "That was another big one as an executive director.... Any small change you make here is going to have huge effects, ripple effects and unintended consequences ... and trying to manage all those things [is difficult]." Half of the interviewees specifically mentioned feeling the weight of the consequences of decisions made.

Another aspect of the job mentioned as creating a sense of pressure was in the area of human resources. A director summed up a stressful aspect by saying, "One of the hardest things for me is when somebody really wants to do the job and they just can't do it and having to fire them or free them up for employment elsewhere." Combining the aspect of terminating employees with managing a budget was also an aspect of the job identified by one director as creating pressure in the job: "So we did restructuring. We laid off 28 positions. Some, six, were vacant. [That was] pretty traumatic for me." This same director went on to say, "There have been many times that I didn't like the job." The pressure of living with the fallout of the decisions one makes, firing employees, laying off employees, and other responsibilities were mentioned by all of the directors. For the interviewees, that weight became something that they had to get to a point of being able to live with if they were to remain in their jobs. This ability to get to a point where one can live with the stress and pressure is a requirement for being able to go forward. One director put it very succinctly,

> And so you really have to be comfortable with your voice, with your face. And to some extent with your relationship, understanding that you are going to be ... people are going to be angry. People are going to dislike you. And [you have to] be okay with that.

Despite coming to grips with the fact that in order to do the job one has to be able to handle and manage the pressure of being the final decision maker and, quite possibly, be disliked by staff, four of the six directors mentioned that there is a sense of aloneness to the job: In other words, as director you do not have any peers. For one director the reality sunk in this way, as she addressed her executive staff,

> And when I got appointed CEO I met with them and said, "You understand now that [our] relationship's going to change. So we can't be buddies anymore." And that was ... that was probably one of the things that was emotionally most difficult.

She went on to say, "But I said, 'I will tell you all one thing; we'll never be friends. So I won't be going to your social gatherings; it's going to be arms' length.' And I told them why, and they understood that." Along with the strongly felt differentiation from the rest of the staff and administration this director also described the sense of always having to keep her guard up at some level. "[I do] not let my guard down. Learning to be very careful about what you say, and consciously not just react [is imperative]." Along with this sense of the need to keep her guard up, the director also described the sense of aloneness in that there was no one between her and the board of directors; in a sense, she was exposed. She explained that this provoked not only a sense of isolation but also one of anxiety,

And I remember thinking to myself, there's no one now between me and the board of directors. I'm out there on my own. I had that buffer before. And the accountability has stepped up several notches. So I was pretty anxiety ridden.

Describing the pressure. This sense of being alone in the job, stemming from having no peers in the organization and from being the person who ultimately has to be responsible for everything that happens, is a heavy burden. It adds to the overall stress and pressure felt by the directors. That stress was described in detail by three of the six directors. One of them stated,

> I'm not a stupid person. I'm trying to ... I'm trying to do the best I can. I really care about our clients and what we're doing. And I care about our staff as much as we can. I care about the system. And I think we're doing a lot of good. But I am really lost, and I'm ... once in a while I have to ... I always have to take walks. I have to take a walk and just remind myself about clients and what's best for clients and [ask] how does that filter out to all these millions of layers?

In describing the difficulties of the amount of intrusion the job has on his life, this same director said,

> There were big pockets of time where it was job, job, job, job, job, job, job. And I did miss some stuff, I forgot or missed some stuff that was really important. I did my best at balancing it, but it wasn't quite good enough. But now that I'm a little bit older and have some friends who have died and some that are in the process now, I still work as hard as I can, but I don't feel guilty when I take a flex day or actually use all my vacation. Still, [I] never take a sick day. If I'm sick, I usually use the flex time or vacation time.

Feeling the pressure. In further explaining the pressure of the job and its intrusion, one director remarked,

> I think [there's a need to] recognize the weight of what you carry. ... and at points, the heaviness of that. And at other points the exuberance that comes with that. Recognize the darks and the lights that come with power. And understand your own response to that, because that's critical in how you're going to interact within and outside the organization.

Another director stated,

And I still feel a lot of that [pressure] inside, I believe: an impossible job to do right. As I said, you can live here in this. And you'd never, ever, ever be able to get it all done. You never.... It's an impossible job.

She continued, "I think most directors, when I talk to them, are feeling fragmented. If I wasn't [not very far] from retirement, I think I might be thinking about a different job in three or four years." In discussing the stress and pressure, yet another director stated that he had learned that to do the job he has to take care of himself.

So both [pressure and stress are an issue], I think [for] anyone in this kind of position, due to the fact there's a lot of stress, especially these days—a lot of stress, a lot of anxiety. It just requires people to be more physically and mentally healthy.

The directors all, in one way or another, then, were deeply aware of their role as protector, the impact that power has on their role, and the pressure they feel as they live out their role as directors. Along with these components of being a director came a fourth element, that of the political realities of the job. The directors I interviewed spoke of how politics, both externally in the industry and in communities they serve and internally with staff, all require them to gain a sense of awareness and skill in order to effectively do their jobs.

Political Realities

The realization that there are political forces they must manage within the industry, community, and agency was a topic that the directors discussed. They acknowledged how important it is that they successfully navigate the political landscape to accomplish their job. They spoke about how they traverse the external politics of their communities, as well as the internal agency politics, in order to move the agency's mission forward.

External politics. The directors discussed external politics very frankly. One, when asked how important a role awareness of politics played, stated, "Being aware is crucial." The directors all clearly identified political influences as a force they had to manage. One director put it this way: "You just have to ... well ... meet politicians. You have to understand what the dynamic is that's helping them make decisions." He spoke of the need to understand the political operatives so that, as a director, one could act in a way, or influence in a way, that benefitted one's organization. This same director described the way he viewed political forces or politicians and how he had internalized the reality so that it could work for him: "You know, you're just joining with people. It's just [that] people are people. And just because they're an elected official, they're not any different than [you]." This director emphasized "joining with" the political forces in a way that allowed his organization to benefit. Another director, on the other hand, discussed the concept of "aligning" with the political forces in a way that created a relationship where both benefit. In the context of discussing how she works with local politicians and bureaucracies she said,

> Alignment. I think the only thing that I would want to add to that would be that alignment, in and of itself, is extraordinarily powerful and has the ability to create opportunities. One must also be very cognizant of when one is not in alignment and cannot be in alignment and make concrete choices about what is your presentation in those instances. When you are saying to another organization or entity, "I can't align with you," what does that look like? Because there is a number of ways that that can look. It can look combative. There's a way to be unaligned-aligned…. And that creates opportunities for you to buy in.

This director further discussed the necessity of being able to work in a political construct when there is the potential from a bureaucracy to harm your organization.

> You [speaking of an outside bureaucracy] see someone who is potentially adversarial or wanting to perhaps take advantage of my organization. There [are] ways I can allow you to buy in and still save face. And I think that that's very important. I think it's [a] very difficult skill set [to learn].

Although both of these directors spoke of the realm of politics and how they manage in a somewhat general way, another director was more specific about

> seeing all the hidden rules that go outside. And if I want to move the agency forward, and I need something from this person, how do I go about doing that? I mean it's a very political world…. And I reached out to our local United Way, who's very savvy on how the community works, and ask[ed] for some help on how … I [should] do this.

This director gave an example, then, of some specific action steps he had taken in order to locate himself and his agency in a place of being joined or aligned, taking into consideration local political forces: "For example, I'm in leadership positions in other nonprofits that aren't like ours, because I feel it's really important to also be a board member some place." This director also cautioned, "Obviously, [though], you have to avoid the conflict of interest." Another director spoke about how she was not only involved in local and community political issues but felt that playing a role in state-wide political issues that related to the community mental health industry was important. "I've always … even prior to becoming a CEO, I've been always active on a lot of statewide committees, a lot of local committees." This director went to describe how she believed that staying politically active through serving on committees and legislative advocacy helps one's organization move its mission forward,

> and if you stay active in your field, I think that plays some of the politics for you, because the more active you are, the more people you need ... and the more you spread tentacles and you're able to advance your ideas or your thoughts or your opinions and hear those of others.

Internal politics. Along with discussing how they navigate the realities of external politics, four of the six directors also discussed how they navigated the internal politics of their organizations in relation to decision making. One director said he uses focus groups to gain a consensus around decisions,

> but I always, like, when I ... when we've got some problem or issue that we need to solve, some systemic kind of thing, when we develop a focus group, and I use focus groups a lot, I always make sure that the majority of the people in that group are the people that are going to have to live with whatever the decision is.

He clarified, in relation to internal politics, how he had discerned when a focus group was helpful: "But on large systemic issues where I believe there's going to be long-term impact, good or bad, then we bring together a focus group."

Another director emphasized the importance of listening to her staff in relation to leading and making decisions. "If you can actually listen to people," she explained, "that's going to give you the head start on any kind of administrative thing." She went on to stay that she uses the practice of listening, "and then, based on that listening, if you can, you know, just show some understanding, some empathy, all those good counseling skills and everything, [you can] use that then to, in a plan-ful way, [help make decisions that have buy in]." Another director mentioned relying internally on a variety of professionals and how the expertise of these individuals helps in decision making.

> [The] CFO's better at the money piece and all. My director of development has much better social skills than I do. And my counsel knows the law better than I do. So, yeah. Yeah, I've got board members who understand different aspects of this business. You know, one's a lobbyist, one's a managing partner of a law firm, and the other one's a banker, and the other one is a businessman. So they each have a skill that I use here that's more polished than the skill I have.... So you surround yourself with ... at least, when I surround myself with competent people or [those] better than I am at what they do, it's great. I learn.

Two other directors discussed the impact of internal politics and how sometimes directors have to make decisions that they believe are best for their agency but that also risk a negative outcome in relation to the internal politics. According to one, "[Regardless of how I feel] I still need to make a decision that's difficult to make." The other director stated, in relation to the internal political environment of the organization, that in reality there are times a decision has to be made and the results or staff reaction lived with regardless of the politics, "and you ... well, if you take your best shot at it and then realize that you can't, you show up the next day and deal with whatever consequences there are."

Finally, one director explained using the internal leadership team and community input to manage decisions and develop an internal culture that helps the agency be successful:

> You can't do it [accomplish the mission of the organization] alone. You are going to have to partner with someone. Ideally, it's your executive team. It needs to be your executive team, as well as individuals in the community, for the greater good. So, the inclusionary piece is very important.

Political skills, both external and internal, therefore are a critical piece to doing the job of being an executive director of a community mental health center. The interviewees identified being able to navigate local and state politics as essential to the overall success of the mission. They also noted that being aware of and sensitive to the internal politics of their organization was key. Most of the internal political skill was described as essential to decision making and creating a culture that assisted in accomplishing the mission; but another theme that emerged from the information provided in the interviews and mentioned by all six interviewees involved self-awareness, genuineness, and seeking feedback. These three traits are aspects of leaders that fit into the authentic leadership framework (Avolio & Gardner, 2005; Gardner et al., 2005; Luthans & Avolio, 2003; Walumbwa et al., 2008), and therefore this theme is identified in this paper as *authentic leadership*.

Authentic Leadership

Self-awareness. All six of the directors identified a strong sense of self-awareness. They were also able to discuss how this self-awareness allowed them to temper their personalities to be more effective as leaders. Four of the directors remarked that they have strong personalities and that they have to be careful to temper them to avoid tamping down the ideas and opinions of others. One director stated, "[I have] an awareness of why some people get intimidated by me. So [I] try to ratchet it down a little bit." Another director with similar personality traits said,

I'm a very controlling personality. And I try to keep that in check most of the time, but it slips out.... I'm so competitive and so driven that I tend to over-dominate people. And then they ... they don't feel good about me. So it's something I try to keep in my awareness all the time.

The two other directors acknowledged that, rather than needing to be aware of a strong overbearing personality, they had to keep other aspects of themselves in mind in order to lead and be their best. One stated,

I think what I learned about myself here is that I need to really keep in mind constantly my own personal strengths and weaknesses so that I don't get caught in the quagmire of what's going on around me.

A second example of awareness offered by an interviewee was

I know that I'm the type of person who can, for the good of whatever the objective is out there, ... I can put aside my personal whatever and work towards some kind of common ... or some sort of consensus or some sort of way to get the objective done.

Yet a third example, cited also as an example of growing pains, was the following:

What else I learned about myself was that I have a tendency to be very empathetic to anybody's pain all the time. And I've learned that [there are] certain times that I can still feel the empathy, but I still need to make a decision that's difficult to make.

Genuineness. Along with the aspect of self-awareness, three of the six interviewed directors identified the necessity of being genuine in their conduct as a key factor in their leadership style. One director declared the necessity to

try to be who I am no matter who I'm with.... And you can be blunt and say, "I don't know what the hell I'm doing now," ... but in general, I think people can feel more valuable if they feel more a part of the process. And so, I guess I need to find new ways to help them feel that they really are a part of the process and not just doing what the boss wants them to do.... People like to know that they've been heard. They like to know their ideas are being considered, even if [they] can't be enacted. And that, in and of itself, I think, sometimes helps to facilitate a smoother process.

Another director explained how she let genuineness and a sincere desire to listen to others assist her in leading effectively:

> I'm not somebody that lets a lot of petty things get in the way. And I'm not somebody who has to impose my will over all else.... I'm willing to listen to all points of view, and I'll sort it out and come to the best decision possible.... And I think it's just important to let the other party or the other person know that she or he has been heard ... and that you're willing to work with anyone involved in any kind of situation or initiative in an equal, participatory kind of fashion. And I think that's really important. Because I think that people perceive, for the most part, when you're not trying to set a hierarchy. Yeah. I rarely even ... I rarely even call people my staff or whatever. It's just people I work with.

This director went on to say how this genuine approach helps her manage disagreements,

> But I think part of being that CEO or director or whatever also is being able to demonstrate, "Yes, I listened and the answer still has to be no," and explaining why the reason might be. And I think it is something ... I think that your position has some merit when you talk to whoever. But being able to demonstrate, you know, some course of action after that, listening ... or to direct a further conversation or to dig deeper into what maybe that person is thinking about.

Another director discussed the importance of a genuine approach in dealing with staff and how it impacts his leadership: "But being fair and equitable and consistent [is important]. Always following through with what you say you're going to do. Even though there have been times ... I mean, I've had to do things that I just hated to have to do." Finally, another interviewee discussed the aspect of genuineness by which he empowers the staff,

> I always knew I had a very strong tendency towards affirmation; I moved into this position, and I became very aware that that was very strongly balanced by accountability.... And there is no weakness in having a leader stand up and say what we are doing is nothing short of transformative. You work miracles everyday.... Because my belief is that the leaders need to. To be an effective leader, we need to do so with as minimal of our own ego as can be involved.

Seeking feedback. The third aspect of authentic leadership that the interviews revealed was the importance of feedback. Three of the six interviewees gave strong examples of how they viewed the importance of feedback in their leadership experience. One stated how important she felt it was in her leadership style, "and in my mind it's perfectly okay for people to disagree with me and say, 'You're nuts, and let's find a different way to do this.'" Another director stated it this way:

> Yeah, you've got to have objective feedback. You've got to have that feedback loop. 'Cause I mean your spouse tells you you're great most of the time…. I try to make it really easy for people [at work] to give me negative feedback, whether that be my peers or that be people here. Whether that negative feedback is accurate or not, it's all good feedback. And it's good feedback to know the areas in which I can improve.

Another director spoke of how important an open door policy is, as well as creating an environment that allows for all employees to give feedback,

> And, you know, people—new employees—know that I have an open-door policy or an open e-mail policy, whatever they're comfortable with. You know, some people are comfortable, they can walk in and sit down and ask me a question and talk to me. Some are more comfortable with the distance of e-mail but by saying to them, if they're not getting answers from their supervisor or supervisor's supervisor, then, "Come to me. I've got nothing to hide. You want to see the finances? Here, have a look," you know, it's just all there. They were also people that would give me good feedback about me. And I've always told staff, "Don't be afraid of me. You can come to me with anything." And of course not very many people [take] me up on that, but there are a few that are comfortable enough with themselves that [will] tell me what I don't want to hear.

The directors I interviewed reflected aspects of self-awareness, genuineness, and seeking feedback about their performance. They felt that these attributes were important for them to be able to perform their jobs at the highest level. Self-awareness provided the insight necessary to adapt to the needs of their staff. Genuineness allowed the leaders to listen to staff more effectively and make fair-minded decisions. Finally, by seeking feedback the directors were able to create an environment where staff felt safe bringing forward their thoughts which, in turn, strengthened the organization.

Practicing Self-Care

The final theme that emerged from the interviews was the importance of self-care. Four of the six directors discussed the importance of taking care of themselves both physically and emotionally.

The subthemes found within the components of both becoming a director and being a director indicate that the director's job creates both physical and mental challenges for the interviewees. To stay in the job long term, four of those interviewed indicated that taking care of themselves on a regular basis was absolutely necessary. Of the four, the first discussed self-care from the perspective of allowing himself to make mistakes and not being too hard on himself or taking himself too seriously:

> There are going to be some big huge mess-ups, sometimes, that you can either worry about or fixate about ... and ... drive yourself nuts. Or you can put everything back together that needs to be there and take it as a learning lesson: How do we avoid this from happening again? Because otherwise I think you can drive yourself nuts.

Another director talked about the importance of having a good support system outside of work.

> But I think a part of that is, too, getting what I need outside the office so that I come in a hundred percent, having really good ... again, a different support system than my professional one ... but a support system where I have good healthy relationships outside of the office so that I'm not trying to get some of my needs for friendship or companionship fulfilled here at the office.

A third director emphasized the importance of physical fitness,

> And to have the stamina to do [the job] and do it reasonably well, I've had to make sure that I am reasonably physically fit. So, from a health standpoint, you know, I keep an eye on my physical health pretty closely ... and [my] mental health, as well. I've learned over the years that physical exercise is good for your mental health too; it keeps your mind alert.

As was cited before in regard to feeling the pressure of the job, a fourth director emphasized the need to get away for both physical and mental well-being.

> But I don't feel guilty when I take a flex day or actually use all my vacation. Still, [I] never take a sick day. If I'm sick, I usually use the flex time or vacation time. [By doing that] what I'm doing ... [is] that I am going to lose myself for a while and not have any balance. And there's no way to do this job, I don't think, without doing that sometimes.

The importance of self-care described by these four directors indicates that in order to do the job of a director one must be vigilant in assuring that time is set aside relationally, emotionally, mentally, and physically to rejuvenate. They highlighted that it is important not to take oneself too seriously and to be able to learn from mistakes rather than being too self-critical. These factors, along with having a good support network, exercising, and taking time away, all contribute to being able to stand up to the rigors of the job.

These six subthemes: filling the role of protector, accepting the impact of power, feeling the pressure, understanding political realities, leading with authenticity, and practicing self-care, comprise the phenomenon of *being a director* of a community mental health center after beginning one's career as a clinician. As protector, the participants discussed protecting the mission, staff and business of their agencies. They also described detailed aspects of the power within the job, such as feeling the weight of the power, having the final say, suffering the consequences of acting on their power, and often feeling as though they do not have power. The participants described the pressure they felt and the aspects of their job that it comes from, as well as the political realities of their work and the importance of successfully navigating external and internal political forces. Characterizing their leadership style by being authentic through self-awareness, genuineness, and seeking feedback, along with the importance of practicing self-care, made up the final two subthemes for *being a director*. The two major themes of *being a director* and *becoming a director,* along with the subthemes found in each, provide the detailed picture used to answer the primary research question.

Conclusion

In summary, the interviews conducted with the six community mental health center executive directors who transitioned into their jobs after beginning as clinicians yielded information that assists in describing a developmental process within the clinician-to-director experience. The data from the interviews produced two overarching themes. The first theme relates to data that centered around the experience of *becoming a director*. Within this theme were seven subthemes: The directors described (a) an organic developmental process that could not necessarily be viewed as either linear or cyclical; (b) an identification of administrative skills developed early on in their careers as clinicians; (c) the attainment, during their transition, of an expanded view of the world in which they worked; (d) the impact of many people along the way who helped shape and mold them as administrators; (e) growing savvy in dealing with people and relationships; (f) a process of transition which included painful experiences that yielded personal and professional growth and understanding; and (7) the necessity, in the end, of changing their view of themselves and embracing an identity that included being the executive director of an agency.

The second overarching theme centers around data that described the phenomenon of *being a director*. Six subthemes that made up this theme were (a) the role of being the protector of the agency, which involves protecting the mission, the persons served, and the staff; (b) the reality of the power of the job and its impact on the organization, the staff, and the director; (c) the pressure felt by directors while experiencing their job; (d) the importance of successfully managing external and internal politics; (e) the effort to remain authentic as a leader; and (f) the importance of self-care to sustain themselves in the job.

One director, in concluding thoughts about the scope of the job and the impact on self, as well as on staff and people served, summed up the interview this way:

> There is no magic. There is only leadership, and … you give definition to what that looks like. And for us it's an embracing of ideas and then a final voice ... but the magic is, you know, opening the ears to the voices and to letting people experience hearing their own voices.

In Chapter V of this dissertation, I will look at how the data gathered from the interviews relate to information contained in the literature review. In particular, I will compare the findings to the adult development and adult learning theories and the theories of leadership development found in Chapter III.

CHAPTER V

Conclusions and Recommendations

The purpose of this phenomenological study was to gain an in-depth understanding of the process of leadership development of individuals who entered the mental health field as clinicians and moved into executive director positions at community mental health centers. By completing the study I hoped to add to the field of mental health administration information that would assist in enhancing executive leadership development in the future. The study was designed to answer one primary and three secondary questions. The primary question was, What is the developmental experience of CMHC directors who begin their careers as clinicians and become effective executive directors? The three sub-questions were as follows: (a) What do CMHC directors describe as the most helpful resources during this transitional process? (b) What are the most important lessons those directors have learned through those resources? (c) What competencies did the directors consider to be most important for them to learn?

The reason for focusing on those four questions is to create an understanding of how successful directors have matured in their careers. It is my hope that understanding this phenomenon will give others who are working to develop inexperienced or new mental health agency directors into effective leaders insight into the process involved in the maturation of the leaders-in-training. Specifically, understanding how successful mental health agency leaders have learned to do their job will provide insight into the kinds of activities or experiences that are needed to train new leaders. These insights also may be helpful in crafting a leadership training model for future CMHC executive directors.

The study consisted of interviewing six executive directors of community mental health centers in Ohio who had begun their careers as clinicians. Each director completed two interviews, the first a structured interview focusing on 14 specific questions (see Appendix A) and the second a more open-ended interview and follow-up questions.

In this concluding chapter, I will (a) discuss the outcomes and present how the findings of the study presented in the previous chapter relate to the primary research question and the three sub-questions, (b) discuss how the findings relate to the theories on leadership development presented in the literature review, (c) discuss the implication of the findings on the practice of community mental health leadership, (d) discuss potential areas for future research, and (f) provide personal reflection on my experience with the research process and the meaning of the data.

Outcomes

Findings for the Primary Research Question

The primary research question for this study is, What is the developmental experience of CMHC directors who begin their careers as clinicians and become effective executive directors?

The data in this study indicated that community mental health center executive director development progressed in two broad stages. The first stage was a period of "becoming a director" followed by reaching the point of "being a director." These two broad developmental steps were made up of several subcomponents that detailed the meaning of each phase.

The stage of becoming a director consisted of seven facets, undergoing an organic developmental process that was unique based on one's life experiences; having others identify leadership skills and abilities early on in one's career and then beginning to develop those skills; gaining an expanded perspective (worldview) of the realm of community mental health and what is involved in accomplishing the task of running a center; being impacted by various people along the way, including peers, board members, supervisors, community and family members; growing savvy in managing various relationships and political situations; experiencing difficult times that create stress and anxiety related to being in charge; and finally, experiencing a shift in identity from feeling overwhelmed and inadequate or new in the job to embracing the role of being the leader of the organization.

The stage of being a director was comprised of six subcomponents. The first subcomponent was living out the role of protector for the agency. Aspects of this role were protecting the mission of the agency, protecting the staff, and protecting the business. The next subcomponent was understanding the impact the power of the job has on a director. The four facets of this second subcomponent included the weight of power, the responsibility of having the final say on all decisions, the consequences of using power, and finally, the perceived absence of power. The third aspect of being a director was identified as feeling the pressures of the job. Two sources of pressure discussed were the need to make major decisions for the organization and the need to deal with various human resource issues, and for this last category the directors also described the pressure and how that pressure felt.

The fourth component of being a director was dealing with the political realities of the industry. The interviewees discussed the political forces they had to deal with as coming from both outside their organization, such as community and industry politics, and within, such as internal politics related to staff and internal relationships. The fifth element of being a director that surfaced from the interviews was being an authentic leader. The directors discussed three aspects of this component: being self-aware, being genuine, and seeking feedback. The final element of being a director was understanding the importance of practicing self-care. The data reflected the importance of mental, relational, and physical wellness in doing the job of executive director.

Theoretical Correlations

Becoming a director. The theoretical framework on which this study was built was adult development and adult learning. This framework was then used as the foundation for how I analyzed the data.

The first subtheme that emerged under the primary theme of becoming a director was that those interviewed had experienced an organic growth process that was specific to each individual. The interviewees described being impacted in their process by various people such as family, teachers, other professionals, or supervisors they had encountered along the way toward becoming a director. This multifaceted and individualized experience can be understood by considering Bronfenbrenner's (1979, 1989; see also Bronfenbrenner et al., 1986) ecological systems model. Bronfenbrenner explained that people's lives and behavior are influenced by several layers of society from the most intimate and immediate, one's family, to the more remote greater cultural beliefs and systems. This model, which is explained in further detail in Chapter II of this dissertation, allows for a way to conceptualize the many factors that impact the development of an individual who begins his or her mental health career as a clinician and moves into the role of being an executive director.

The second subcomponent to becoming a director found in the study was early identification of administrative skills. The interviewees all had held management and supervisory positions before they became executive directors. They had been placed in these roles because other leaders in the field identified them as having management and administrative skills. Although this identification at first may seem subjective, clear competencies that are involved in leading were noticeably stronger in some clinicians than in others. Gardner (1990) discussed several tasks that make up the act of leadership. One of the tasks he identified is "managing" (Gardner, 1990, p. 14). He described management as consisting of planning, prioritizing, organizing, building institutional frameworks, keeping the system functions, setting agendas, making decisions, and exercising political judgment. Excelling in these management tasks seems to be the earliest identifier for clinicians who were placed on the track to becoming administrators.

The third component of the theme of becoming a director, having an expanded worldview, has been discussed by several authors (e.g., Argyris & Schön, 1974; Bateson, 1972; Watzlawick, Weakland, & Fisch, 1974) in relation to adult development and learning. The interviewees acknowledged that this expanded worldview moved them from regarding the work in community mental health as entailing one-on-one interactions with persons served to a broader understanding of the financial, regulatory, political, and human resource factors involved in operating a community mental health center. Bateson (1972) described this type of learning as level II learning, in which "we learn about and classify the context in which learning takes place" (as cited in Bale, 1992, p. 19). Another adult learning theory that coincides with the expanded worldview experience is Watzlawick, Weakland, and Fisch's (1974) second-order change. As the directors in this present study moved from working as clinicians and only viewing the operations from a clinical perspective to adopting a person-served perspective and began to see the work from a much broader vantage point, they began adapting their view from the originally established framework, as is reflected by the work of Watzlawick et al. (1974) and also that of Bartunek and Moch (1987). The concept of double-loop learning (Argyris & Schön, 1974) is also comparable to this expanded worldview, as this type of learning involves questioning one's original beliefs about a problem and then adapting new values and understanding about it. Such learning was evidenced when the participating interviewees identified how prior to being directors they had perceived the primary problems as getting paperwork done and being effective in one-on-one counseling relationships. With their expanded worldview, they now see how the work done with persons served connects to the financial well-being of the agency.

In regard to the fourth subcomponent of becoming a director, the impact of people, the interviewees identified various people both inside and outside their professional lives who had influenced them along the way. This component of the development is supported in Bronfenbrenner's (1979, 1989; see also Bronfenbrenner et al., 1986) concept of microsystems within his ecological systems theory. The microsystem involves a person's thoughts and behaviors being influenced by "a pattern of activities, roles, and interpersonal relations experienced by the developing persons in a given setting with particular physical and material characteristics" (Bronfenbrenner, 1979, p. 22). Those interviewed for this study explained how co-workers and supervisors, family members, and even former college professors had influenced them. These members of the microsystem helped the participants change their behavior to both more like and less like that of the people they were encountering.

The fifth aspect of becoming a director, "becoming savvy," is about the directors' learning to manage different types of relationships, whether with individuals, communities, or political entities. Piaget and Inhelder (1969) used their theory of cognitive development to describe how this happens. Those authors discussed the concept of "schemes" (Piaget & Inhelder, 1969, p. 7), which are the basic structures of information people have that make up how they understand life and the world around them. When new information is taken in, people have to either absorb it and adapt their scheme so that what they know includes the new information or reject the new data because that information does not make sense with what they already know. As directors experience new realties in regard to what it means to operate a mental health center, including managing the relationships they encounter, they are adapting their old scheme to include the new information.

Bandura (2004) also discussed how people can reflect on what they experience and alter what they believe in order to include the new information. He described four sources of information through which people adapt their behavior, "performance attainment; vicarious experiences of observing the performances of others; verbal persuasion and allied types of social influences that one possesses certain capabilities [*sic*]; and physiological states from which people partly judge their capabilities, strength, and vulnerability" (p. 41). The present interviewees who described how their experiences helped them become more knowledgeable and perceptive had become so by learning through the four sources identified by Bandura. For instance, when the directors in this study described learning about how to address human resource issues such as hiring or firing staff, they mentioned learning this by having personal successes or failures with these tasks. Along with learning by direct experience, at least two of the directors spoke specifically about vicarious learning as they described seeing previous directors do the job poorly or in ways that created an unpleasant work environment and how those observations led them to change their behavior. In addition to direct experience and vicarious learning, one director, in particular, discussed how verbal persuasion helped him learn that he had made good choices in regard to managing underperforming staff. He discussed the positive feedback he received from employees in the agency when he took a stand and fired workers that others considered unethical. Finally, the participating interviewees described the feeling of pressure and stress that was associated with being the final decision maker for their organizations. This sense of pressure and stress, stemming from the importance and isolation of their decision making role, caused them to question and judge their capabilities, strength, and vulnerability.

The sixth component of becoming a director was experiencing growing pains. The directors discussed feeling anxiety caused by the weight of their responsibility, as well as learning by experiencing difficulties. This element of the learning process is reflected in the research of McKenna, Boyd, and Yost (2007), who found in their research sample of pastors that 32% of the "[leadership] development experiences occurred in the trenches" (p. 179), and 27% occurred in "times of transition" (p. 179). Similarly, Bennis and Thomas (2002) discussed "the crucibles of leadership" (p. 87), identifying a process by which leaders emerge from the period of testing better able to lead.

The last factor in the theme of becoming a leader was experiencing an identity shift, from being a clinician to embracing the role of executive director. This subtheme described the directors' struggles to embrace the reality that they were in charge: that they were responsible and that the agency was in their command. Although the research presented in Chapter II of the present study does not speak directly to the phenomenon of an identity shift, Amey (2005) described a model of development in which leaders move from seeing leadership as primarily a top-down enterprise to becoming more inclusive to being more servant-like. Boyatzis (1999) and Goleman, Boyatzis, and McKee (2002) discussed the process by which leaders develop into their ideal selves. The identity shift phenomenon experienced by the present interviewees is similar in that the interviewees evolved into more mature and sophisticated leaders although not identifying as their "ideal self" per se.

In Chapter II of this dissertation, I discussed the change process in leadership development. The experience of becoming a director as described by the present interviewees is, in effect, a change process. A review of the theories presented in this particular section of Chapter II reveals that the theorists related to the phenomenon of becoming a director in the following ways. First, Amey (2005) stated in her cognitive process model that "leadership involves cognitive processes, meaning-making for self and others, and has a developmental orientation" (p. 690). Five of the six directors interviewed for the present research study did feel that there was a personal change process involved in transitioning from clinician to director. The work-experience model reflected in the research of Bennis and Thomas (2002) and of McKenna, Yost, and Boyd (2007) also described how work experience assists leaders in gaining the skills and understanding that they need to do a more effective job. In agreement with Bennis and Thomas's (2002) work on the "crucibles of leadership" (p. 87) model and McKenna, Yost, and Boyd's (2007) finding that a large part of leadership learning occurs "in the trenches" (p. 179), the directors involved in this dissertation research were all able to discuss how their work experience has helped them be more effective in handling problems and responsibilities in their jobs. Boyatzis (1999) and Goleman et al. (2002) discussed the process by which leaders develop into their ideal selves. An example of this component of the developmental process was when the directors in this study described transitioning from being unable to embrace the identity of executive director to the point at which they were able to embrace the role. In doing so they were manifesting a more mature and effective form of themselves as leaders. Lastly, Quinn, Spreitzer, and Brown (2000) developed the advanced change model, which describes 10 steps leaders move through to eventually evolve to the point of becoming focused on the greater good and impacting the greater system around them. Demonstrating Quinn et al.'s final step of focusing on impacting the system for the greater good, two of the directors in particular discussed becoming frustrated with the political forces that often act in ways that do not benefit some of the most vulnerable people their agencies serve. They worked at finding ways to redirect the political forces and impact the system in a way that benefited those vulnerable individuals.

Being a director. The second primary theme in the present research was identified as that of being a director. This theme had six subthemes: (a) being in the role of protector of the agency's mission, staff, and business; (b) dealing with the impact of power, including the weight of power, the power of having the final say, the consequences of power, and the perceived absence of power; (c) experiencing the pressure of the job; (d) understanding the realities of both internal and external politics; (e) striving to be authentic in their role as leaders; and (f) practicing self-care.

The first subtheme was being in the role of protector. This theme entailed protecting the mission of the organization, protecting the staff, and protecting the business aspects of the agency. Gardner (1990) discussed several roles that leaders take on that define leadership. He mentioned the need for leaders to protect the mission by engaging in "perpetual rebuilding" (p. 13) in order to protect the organization from having its values "decay over time" (p. 13). He also described leaders as having the responsibility of envisioning goals and affirming their organization's values (pp. 12–13). The directors I interviewed spoke of the need to do such reaffirming of values in several ways. One way was by weeding out staff who did not behave in ways consistent with the organization's values. They also spoke of the need to make decisions consistent with being fiscally responsible, so that the business could go on accomplishing its mission. One director, in particular, discussed the need to provide for the self-care of the staff who are regularly victims of secondary trauma.

The next subtheme, dealing with the power inherent in the job, entailed the executive directors describing their experience with the power that rests in the job. They discussed feeling the weight of the power, having the final say in important agency matters, managing the reality that their use of power can and often does have strong consequences, and finally, knowing that despite having power they often see their directives not done the way they wanted or unheeded. One director perceptively stated, "Just because I am the boss doesn't make them believe me." Another director shared her insight when she said, "The only real way to get people to do want you want is to get them to buy into you." As discussed in Chapter II, Burns (1978), in his work describing transformational leadership, has stated that "inducing followers to act for certain goals that represent the values and motivations—the wants and needs, the aspirations and expectations—of both leaders and followers" (p. 19) aligns with the use of power in a way that helps others buy in. Bass (1985) further discussed transformational leadership as motivating others past their self-interest toward doing actions for the good of the organization; this type of leadership wields power in a way that strengthens others and the organization. As one director put it, "Power now is something that is light. It's transformative. It's translucent. It's something that helps one grow."

The third subtheme under becoming a director involved the pressure inherent with the job. This pressure related to several things, including an awareness of the impact decisions have on people's lives, the need to fire or lay off staff, a sense of aloneness, the time demands of the job, and the number of components to the job. This pressure was described by McKenna, Yost, and Boyd (2007) as "developmental experiences occur[ing] in the trenches" (p. 179), a pressure which, according to Bennis and Thomas (2002) and their concept of "crucibles of leadership" (p. 87), leads to "adaptive capacity" and manifests itself in the qualities of hardiness, learning skills, and creativity (p. 91). Although living with the types of pressures they described may have helped the present directors develop as leaders, they also indicated that the discomfort of the pressure never left. It was a reality of the job of being an executive, and learning to live with it was an integral part of the job.

Dealing with politics, both external and internal, was the fourth subtheme. The interviewees discussed the importance of being aware not only of the impact external politics have on agencies at both the local and state level but also of the importance of being politically active, whether on a local community board or at the state level through the trade association. One of the most powerful external concepts advanced, that of "alignment," came from a director who described the importance of finding ways to be "unaligned-aligned" and remain aligned with political forces in ways that do not sacrifice the agency's mission and also do not destroy an important political relationship. Internally, thus, it is important to develop consensus around big decisions or agency initiatives.

Bandura (2004) discussed the interaction of persons and their environment as having bidirectional influence. In other words, persons influence their environment through their various behaviors and personal factors at the same time that the environment influences them and their reactions or behaviors. This bidirectional interaction of persons and their environment is a factor in how leaders manage both the external and the internal political forces with which they contend. The leader seeks to have an impact with the political forces in a way that helps accomplish the mission of the organization while at the same time benefiting the political faction. The concept of alignment that this one director identified could be explained as a manifestation of this bidirectional influence in which each side's position is strengthened or supported in some way by the other's.

The fifth subtheme that emerged involved the interviewees' mutual sense that striving to be reflexive, genuine, and willing to seek feedback from others was an important characteristic of their leadership style. These characteristics are major components of the authentic leadership model explained by Luthans and Avolio (2003); Avolio and Gardner (2005); Gardner, Avolio, Luthans, May, and Walumbwa. (2005); and Walumbwa, Avolio, Gardner, Wernsing, and Peterson (2008). All interviewees identified an awareness of their personalities and styles of relating to others. They were cognizant of aspects of their personalities that they needed to manage in order to be successful. They also echoed the concern expressed by Argyris (1991) that they might, due to their style or personality, define difficulties or challenges in ways that perpetuate the problem. The interviewees expressed a desire to use this awareness to temper their actions and responses in ways that were of the greatest benefit to the organization and its staff. Some also acknowledged the importance of being able to receive feedback from their coworkers and others concerning how their actions are impacting the organizations. Luthans and Avolio (2003) identified one of the five characteristics of authentic leaders as "remaining cognizant of their own vulnerabilities and openly discussing them with associates so the leader can be questioned to ensure that the direction they [sic] are heading is 'right'" (p. 248). Being genuine, as one director expressed it, "trying to be who I am no matter who I am with," also was a component of being authentic that some of the interviewees discussed. Again, Luthans and Avolio identified this as a key characteristic of an authentic leader, as they stated that "authentic leaders try to operate with no gap (or at least try to constantly narrow the gap) between espoused values (i.e., their true self) and values in action" (p. 248).

The final subtheme associated with the primary theme of becoming a director is practicing self-care. Four of the interviewed directors discussed the importance of taking care of themselves physically, emotionally, and relationally. These four directors all indicated that the job of executive director was very demanding and could encroach in an unhealthy way into one's personal life and physical well-being. They indicated that a director who wanted to stay in the job a long time had to develop a system of self-care. Argyris (1991) expressed a concern that people in general focus on remaining in control, winning, suppressing negative feelings, and making a rational pursuit of objectives. These aspects of one's approach to life, according to the present interviewees, must be tempered in order to remain successful in the job over a long period of time.

The primary research question, What is the developmental experience of CMHC directors who begin their careers as clinicians and become effective executive directors? as viewed through this research project is answered through two principal themes. The first, *becoming a director,* presents the experiences of the directors interviewed who described their journey from beginning their jobs as executive directors until they embraced the full identity of being an executive director. The second theme, *being a director,* presents the ongoing experience of living out the job on a day-to-day basis, detailing the competencies and struggles of the position. The next section will discuss how the data from the interviews respond to the sub-questions, What do CMHC directors describe as the most helpful resources during this transitional process? What are the most important lessons the interviewed directors have learned through those resources? and What competencies did the directors consider to be most important to learn?

Sub-Questions

(1) What do CMHC directors describe as the most helpful resources during this transitional process?

The directors had varying answers as to what was the most helpful resource during the clinician-to-director transition. Their responses included people whom they worked with, failure and risk, and observing bad examples, which showed them what not to do. When interviewees were asked what resource had helped them the most during their transition to director, the predominant answer was people they had encountered along the way. Some directors spoke of their board members as being the most supportive and influential resource; others mentioned staff and members of the management teams with specific duties, such as the chief financial officer or the human resource supervisor. In their research with pastors, McKenna, Yost, and Boyd (2007) found that only 23% of their respondents felt that personal relationships were the context in which they had "developmental experiences" (p. 179). The difference in this dynamic between the pastors in the research presented by McKenna, Yost, and Boyd and the interviewees in this present study who indicated that the greatest resource was relationships may be the relative difference in the nature of pastoral work and being the executive director of a community mental health center. Another factor may be that the executive directors interviewed may work with a much larger staff and have individuals who provide more specific professional supports to them than pastors typically do.

(2) What are the most important lessons the interviewed directors have learned through those resources?

Five of the six directors spoke empathically about how when they were working as clinicians, their view of the business of community mental health was incomplete. The directors spoke of their lessons learned throughout the interview, and those lessons are discussed or identified in the subthemes that encompass the larger themes of becoming a director and being a director. Learning to see the big picture, making wise fiscal decisions, handling human resource problems, dealing with political forces, handling conflict, and responding to problems and failures are all important lessons that the directors identified.

(3) What competencies did the directors consider to be most important to learn?

The competencies the directors felt were important for them are again reflected as subthemes of the two major themes. Being skilled in agency finances, human resources, political factors, problem solving, and decision making were the primary competencies emphasized. These competencies align with Gardner's (1990) tasks of leadership as envisioning goals, affirming values, motivating, managing, achieving workable unity, explaining, serving as a symbol, representing the group, and renewing.

Implications of the Findings on the Practice of
Community Mental Health Leadership

In the beginning of this dissertation I set out to tell the story of the developmental process of community mental health center (CMHC) directors who began their careers as clinicians. Because this is a qualitative study and was not designed to reflect a statistical relevance to the phenomenon, the implication for practice will be based on the belief that the story of the six interviewees has many similarities with the experience of other executive directors who began their careers as clinicians. As I stated in Chapter I, based on the input of the Associate Director of The Ohio Council of Behavioral Health & Family Services Providers, there is an impending crisis of qualified leaders in the field of community mental health. It may be possible to use the information in this study to create a model for leadership training based on the subthemes of the data. As the interviews indicated, the process of development was an individualized experience and not necessarily linear, but there were common experiences. The interviewees indicated that they had been labeled early on in their careers as having administrative potential. Thus it may be feasible to flag for a training program clinicians who are currently in the field and have administrative potential. The program could use the subthemes as modules to help the clinicians develop skills in practical areas such as financial management, human resource best practices, problem solving, and strategic planning. The second phase of the training could help make the directors aware of their role of protecting the mission, understanding and navigating political forces, and practicing effective problem solving and decision making, as well as following a stress management and self-care regime. In a final phase, the new directors could be paired up with experienced directors who would mentor them for one to two years and help them transition less painfully or more efficiently by offering advice and making sense of the new directors' experiences.

Directions for Future Research

This phenomenological study explored the developmental experience of six executive directors of community mental health centers in Ohio who began their careers as clinicians. Although not statistically generalizable, the research may help the field of mental health leadership toward an understanding of what leadership development looks like. I would like to suggest three avenues for future research as a way to gain an even more in-depth understanding of this experience. First is the need to expand the research sample to include a much larger number of directors. Such an expansion would allow for comparison of the present study results with those of the larger sample to develop an even more robust set of common themes.

A second direction for future research would be to complete a qualitative study on two groups of clinicians who moved into the role of executive director, with one group being those who were successful and another group made up of those who left the role after experiencing failure and/or determining the job was not a good fit. Comparing the stories of these two cohorts might reveal what can be done early on in the careers of clinicians who become executive directors to help them be successful. It might also help develop a set of characteristics that make for a successful experience versus an unsuccessful one.

The third area that I would suggest for future research is a gender-separated study involving groups of clinicians who have become executive directors. Although in this present study I did not pursue the identification of differences in the development experience of the interviewees based on gender, this expanded approach would allow for a comparison of the differing experiences between men and women in order to tailor future training programs or mentorships to their specific needs.

A fourth approach for future research would be to do an expanded study developing one of the subthemes. For instance, a study could focus on the phenomenon of developing political skill, and a series of questions be constructed to help draw out the story of how various directors have found that skills sets develop.

Reflections Regarding the Study

My interest in completing this study came from my own experience of beginning my career in community mental health as a clinician, then moving into a supervisory role and eventually becoming an executive. I found myself identifying with the present interviewees and their stories. Some of them are executive directors of much larger agencies than the one at which I work. Some are highly accomplished business people and have transformed their agencies into multimillion dollar corporations. Others serve in smaller organizations and do so with great passion and skill. I learned from all of them. The interviews helped me validate my story and the stress and sometimes painful experiences I have had along the way.

The characteristics described by the present interviewees in their stories mirror many of my own experiences. Like the interviewees for this study, I was informed by one of my supervisors that I had administrative skills. From there I began the role of a clinical supervisor and program director before becoming an executive director. Just as the interviewees described their course of development as nonlinear, I would say my experience could be seen not as linear but rather as an organic process that is still going on. Like the subjects of this study, I have had to develop a much larger view of what it means to accomplish the mission of the mental health center in which I work. That expanded view involves facilitating teamwork among a large number of people and orchestrating client care that begins with an initial phone call and works its way through to becoming a billable service that must be paid. I have learned human resource law, the importance of reading and understanding financial statements, how to plan carefully and strategically, the importance of managing internal and external politics, and the necessity of self-care. I have had to learn to live with being the final decision maker, with the pressure of success and failure, with feeling alone, and with always having to act in a way that not only protects but also accomplishes the agency's mission and business goals while helping the staff do the same. I strive to be authentic and transformational as a leader, but my own humanity often leads me to stumble and struggle with both goals.

The similarities that I found between myself and the research participants are identified as a limitation of this research study. One of the primary reasons that I was interested in studying the phenomenon of the developmental experience of clinicians who become executive directors of community mental health centers is that my own experience has been so powerful. Over the course of my eight years leading an agency, I have found myself learning many lessons the hard way, along with frequently being affirmed by the agency's board of directors and experiencing the agency's moving forward. Emotionally, I have vacillated between being so miserable I wanted to be fired to feeling as if I was in the perfect job. In particular, the emotional experiences I have had most likely caused me to not only identify but also possibly over identify with the participants. This over identification may have led to my projecting my own thoughts and feelings onto the participants. In order to mitigate this possibility, the participants were all given the opportunity to read their transcripts and my interpretation of the transcripts. They were asked to provide feedback in any case in which my interpretation did not match their intent or I was not being accurate in my depiction of their experiences. I also had three peers read the transcripts and the interpretation to ensure that my interpretation was consistent with the information in the interviews. Finally, I reviewed the findings and assessed them for their consistency with other leadership research in the field.

I was fascinated by the fact that the directors, the agencies, and their stories were all different but there were also such similarities in how the directors described both becoming and being directors. Most of all, I was tremendously impressed with the heart of all of the interviewees. Each one is in his or her role because of a desire to help the poor, the traumatized, the homeless, the ones who could easily be described as "the least of these" (Matt. 25:40). I want to thank the six executive directors who allowed me to enter their worlds and to tell their stories with the hope that those stories will live on and help others, the next generation of leaders.

My faith tradition has a story about a Jewish prophet named Jeremiah. He has been chosen by God to lead his people toward a life of faith, morality, justice, and compassion. At one point of frustration, Jeremiah complains about how difficult the job of leading is and that no one cares anymore about the very essential values he is proclaiming. Jeremiah's God replies, "If you have raced with men on foot, and they have wearied you, how will you compete with horses? And if in a safe land you are so trusting, what will you do in the thicket of the Jordan?" (Jer. 12:5). I was reminded of this passage of Scripture as I read through the transcripts of my interviews with the participants in this study. The men and women of this study, every day, are running with horses and moving through the thickets. They are doing their jobs with faith, morality, justice, and compassion. I am thankful for their willingness to share their experiences and to serve the field of community mental health with integrity.

REFERENCES

Allen, S. J. (2007, Spring). Adult Learning Theory & Leadership Development. Kravis Leadership Institute. *Leadership Review, 7,* 26–37.

Allen, W. J. (2001). Chapter 3: The role of action research in environmental management. In *Working together for environmental management: The role of information sharing and collaborative learning.* (Doctoral dissertation). Massey University, New Zealand. Retrieved from http://learningforsustainability.net/ research /thesis/thesis_ch3.html

American Counseling Association. (2005). *ACA Code of Ethics*: Retrieved from http://www.txca.org/Images/tca/Documents/ACA%20Code%20of%20Ethics.pdf

Amey, M. J. (2005). Leadership as learning: Conceptualizing the process. *Community College Journal of Research and Practice, 29,* 689–704. doi: 10.1080 /10668920591006539

Amit, K., Popper, M., Gal, R., Mamane-Levy, T., & Lisak, A. (2009). Leadership-shaping experiences: A comparative study of leaders and non-leaders. *Leadership & Organization Development Journal, 30*(4), 302–318.

Argyris, C. (1991). Teaching smart people how to learn. *Harvard Business Review, 69*(3), 99–109.

Argyris, C., & Schön, D. (1974). *Theory in practice: Increasing professional effectiveness.* San Francisco, CA: Jossey-Bass.

Austin, M. J. (1991). Educating the future mental health administrator. *Administration and Policy in Mental Health, 18*(4), 227–236. doi:10.1007/BF00706047

Avolio, B. J., & Gardner, W. L. (2005). Authentic leadership development: Getting to the root of positive forms of leadership. *The Leadership Quarterly, 16*(3), 315–338. doi:10.1016/j.leaqua.2005.03.001

Baker, S. B., Exum, H. A., & Tyler, R. E. (2002). The developmental process of clinical supervisors in training. *Counselor Education & Supervision, 42*(1), 15–30.

Bale, L. (1992, November). *Gregory Bateson's theory of mind: Practical applications to pedagogy.* [Published online by Lawrence Bale, D&O Press, Nov. 2000]. Retrieved from http://www.narberthpa.com/Bale/lsbale_dop/gbtom_patp.pdf

Bale, L.S. (1995). *Gregory Bateson, cybernetics, and the social/behavioral sciences.* Retrieved from http://www.narberthpa.com/Bale/lsbale_dop/gbcatsbs.pdf

Bandura, A. (1977). *Social learning theory.* New York, NY: General Learning Press.

Bandura, A. (2004). Model of causality in social learning theory. In A. Freeman, M. J. Mahoney, P. DeVito, & D. Martin (Eds.), *Cognition and psychotherapy* (2nd ed., pp. 25–44). New York, NY: Springer.

Barnes, K. L., & Moon, S. M. (2006). Factor structure of the psychotherapy supervisor development scale. *Measurement and Evaluation in Counseling and Development, 39*(3), 130–140.

Bartunek, J. M., & Moch, M. K. (1987). First-order, second-order, and third-order change and organization development interventions: A cognitive approach. *The Journal of Applied Behavioral Science, 23*(4), 483–500. doi: 10.1177/ 002188638702300404

Bass, B. M. (1985). *Leadership and performance beyond expectation.* New York, NY: Free Press.

Bass, B. M., & Avolio, B. J. (1990). The implications of transactional and transformational leadership for individual, team, and organizational development. In W. A. Pasmore & R. W. Woodman (Eds.), *Research in organizational change and development* (4th ed., pp. 231–272). Greenwich, CT: JAI Press.

Bateson, G. (1972). *Steps to an ecology of mind.* New York, NY: Ballantine.

Bennis, W. G., & Thomas, R. J. (2002). *Geeks and geezers: How era, values, and defining moments shape leaders.* Boston, MA: Harvard Press.

Boeree, C. G., (2006). *Erik Erikson.* Retrieved from http://webspace.ship.edu /cgboer/erikson.html

Bergquist, W. (1993). *The post-modern organization: Mastering the art of irreversible change.* San Francisco, CA: Jossey-Bass.

Birren, J. E., & Birren, B. A. (1990). The concepts, models, and history of the psychology of aging. In J. E. Birren & K. W. Schaie (Eds.), *Handbook of the psychology of aging* (3rd ed., pp. 3–20). San Diego, CA: Academic Press.

Boyatzis, R. (1999). Self-directed change and learning as a necessary meta-competency for success and effectiveness in the 21st century. In R. Sims & J. G. Veres (Eds.), *Keys to employee success in the coming decades.* (pp. 15–32). Westport, CT: Greenwood Press.

Bradley, C. L., & Marcia, J. E. (1998). Generativity-stagnation: A five category model. *Journal of Personality, 66*(1), 39-64.

Braun, V., & Clarke, V. (2006). Using thematic analysis in psychology. *Qualitative Research in Psychology, 3*(2), 77–101.

Bronfenbrenner, U. (1979). *The ecology of human development: Experiments by nature and design.* Cambridge, MA: Harvard University Press.

Bronfenbrenner, U. (1989). Ecological systems theory. In R. Vasta (Ed.), *Annals of child development: Vol. 6. Six theories of child development: Revised formulations and current issues* (pp. 187–249). Greenwich, CT: JAI Press.

Bronfenbrenner, U., Kessel, F., Kessen, W., & White, S. (1986). Towards a critical social history of developmental psychology: A propaedic discussion. *American Psychology, 41*(11), 1218–1230.

Buker, B. (2003). Spiritual development and the epistemology of systems theory. *Journal of Psychology and Theology, 31*(2), 143–153.

Burns, J. M. (1978). *Leadership.* New York, NY: Harper & Row.

Caffarella, R. S. (2002). *Planning program for adult learners: A practical guide for educators, trainers, and staff developers.* San Francisco: Jossey-Bass.

Centers for Medicare and Medicaid Services. (n.d.) *Community Mental Health Centers.* Retrieved from http://www.cms.gov/Medicare/Provider-Enrollment-and-Certification/CertificationandComplianc/CommunityHealthCenters.html

Corrigan, P. W., Diwan, S., Campion, J., & Rashid, F. (2002). Transformational leadership and the mental health team. *Administration and Policy in Mental Health, 30*(2), 97–108.

Corrigan, P. W., Garman, A. N., Lam, C., & Leary, M. (1998). What mental health teams want in their leaders. *Administration and Policy in Mental Health, 26*(2), 111–123.

Creswell, J. W. (2007). *Qualitative inquiry and research design choosing: Choosing among five approaches* (2nd ed.). Thousand Oaks, CA: SAGE.

Creswell, J. W. (2009). *Research design: Qualitative, quantitative, and mixed methods approaches* (3rd ed.). Thousand Oaks, CA: SAGE.

Drath, W., & Palus, C. J. (1994). *Making common sense: Leadership as meaning-making in a community of practice.* Greensboro, NC: Center for Creative Leadership.

Dusick, D. M. (2011a). *Bold Educational Software: Writing the assumptions and limitations.* Retrieved from http://bold-ed.com/assumptions.htm

Dusick, D. M. (2011b). *Bold Educational Software: Writing the delimitations.* Retrieved from http://bold-ed.com/delimitations.htm

Eisner, E. W. (1991). *The enlightened eye: Qualitative inquiry and the enhancement of educational practice.* New York, NY: Macmillan.

Erikson, E. H. (1963). *Childhood and society* (2nd ed.). New York, NY: Norton.

Erikson, E. H. (1964). *Insight and responsibility.* New York, NY: Norton.

Erikson, E. H. (1968). *Identity: Youth and crisis.* New York, NY: Norton.

Evans, R. (1996). *The human side of school change: Reform, resistance, and the real-life problems of innovation.* San-Francisco, CA: Jossey-Bass.

Feldman, S. (1973). *The administration of mental health services.* Springfield, IL: Charles C. Thomas.

Feldman, S. (1981). Leadership in mental health: Changing the guard for the 1980's. *Administration in Mental Health, 9*(1), 4–20. doi:10.1007/BF01845808

Foldy, E. G., & Creed, W. E. D. (1999). Action learning, fragmentation, and the interaction of single-, double-, and triple-loop change. *The Journal of Applied Behavioral Science, 35*(2), 207–227. doi:10.1177/0021886399352005

Gardner, J. W. (1990). *On leadership.* New York, NY: Free Press.

Gardner, W. L., Avolio, B. J., Luthans, F., May, D. R., & Walumbwa, F. (2005). "Can you see the real me?" A self-based model of authentic leader and follower development. *The Leadership Quarterly, 16*(3), 343–372. doi:10.1016 /j.leaqua.2005.03.003

Geertz, C. (1973). *The interpretation of cultures.* New York, NY: Basic Books.

Gilligan, C. (1982). *In a different voice.* Cambridge, MA: Harvard University Press.

Glesne, C. (2006). *Becoming qualitative researchers: An introduction* (3rd ed.). Boston, MA: Pearson.

Goleman, D., Boyatzis, R. E., & McKee, A. (2002). *Primal leadership: Learning to lead with emotional intelligence.* Boston, MA: Harvard Business School Press.

Goodman, N. (1984). *Of mind and other matters.* Cambridge, MA: Harvard University Press.

Grusky, O., Thompson, W. A., & Tillipman, H. (1991). Clinical versus administrative backgrounds for mental health administrators. *Administration and Policy in Mental Health, 18*(4), 271–278.

Guba, E. G., & Lincoln, Y. S. (1989). *Fourth generation evaluation.* Newbury Park, CA: SAGE.

Guba, E. G., & Lincoln, Y. S. (1994). Competing paradigms in qualitative research. In N. K. Denzin & Y.S. Lincoln (Eds.), *Handbook of qualitative research* (pp. 105–117). Thousand Oaks, CA: SAGE.

Guba, E.G., & Lincoln, Y.S. (2001). *Guidelines and checklist for constructivist (a.k.a. fourth generation) evaluation.* Retrieved from http://www.wmich.edu/evalctr/archive_checklists/constructivisteval.pdf

Guba, E. G., & Lincoln, Y. S. (2005). Paradigmatic controversies, contradictions, and emerging confluences. In N. K. Denzin & Y.S. Lincoln (Eds.), *The SAGE handbook of qualitative research* (3rd ed., pp. 191–215). Thousand Oaks, CA: SAGE.

Halpern, E. S. (1983). *Auditing naturalistic inquiries: The development and application model.* (Unpublished doctoral dissertation). Indiana University, Bloomington, IN.

Hamachek, D. (1990). Evaluating self-concept and ego status in Erikson's last three psychosocial stages. *Journal of Counseling & Development, 68*(6), 677.

Hawkins, P. (2004). A centennial tribute to Gregory Bateson 1904–1980 and his influence on the fields of organizational development and action research. *Action Research, 2*(4), 409–423. doi:10.1177/1476750304047984

Hirschowitz, R. G. (1971). Dilemmas of leadership in community mental health. *The Psychiatric Quarterly, 45*(1), 102–116. doi:10.1007/BF01574794

Husserl, E. (1970). *The crisis of European sciences and transcendental phenomenology.* Evanston, IL: Northwestern University Press.

Johnson, H. H. (2008). Mental models and transformative learning: The key to leadership development? *Human Resource Development Quarterly, 19*(1), 85–89. doi:10.1002/hrdq.1227

Kegan, R. (2000). What "form" transforms: A constructive-developmental approach to transformative learning. In J. Mezirow (Ed.), *Learning as transformation* (pp. 35–70). San Francisco, CA: Jossey-Bass.

Keshavan, M. (2011). The changing global mental health landscape and need for leadership. *Asian Journal of Psychiatry, 4*(3), 161. doi:10.1016/j.ajp.2011.08.006

Kohlberg, L. (1963). The development of children's orientations toward a moral order. *Vita Humana, 6,* 11–33.

Kohlberg, L. (1969). Stage and sequence: The cognitive developmental approach to socialization. In D. A. Goslin (Ed.), *Handbook of socialization and research.* Chicago, IL: Rand McNally.

Kohlberg. L. (1976). Moral stages and moralization: The cognitive development approach. In T. Lickona (Ed.), *Moral development and behavior: Theory, research and social issues.* New York, NY: Holt, Rinehart, & Winston, CBS College Publishing.

Kotre, J. (1984). *Outliving the self: Generativity and the interpretation of lives.* Baltimore MD: John Hopkins University Press.

Lemme, B. H. (2006). *Development in adulthood* (4th ed.). Boston, MA: Pearson.

Lincoln, Y. S., & Guba, E. G. (1985). *Naturalistic inquiry.* Beverly Hills, CA: SAGE.

Luthans, F., & Avolio, B. (2003). Authentic leadership: A positive development approach. In K. S. Cameron, J. E. Dutton, & R. E. Quinn (Eds.), *Positive organizational scholarship* (pp. 241–258). San Francisco, CA: Berrett-Koehler.

Maslow, A. H. (1943). A theory of human motivation. *Psychological Review, 50*(4), 370–396. doi:10.1037/h0054346

McAdams, D. P., & de St. Aubin, E. (1992). A theory of generativity and its assessment through self-report, behavioral acts, and narrative themes in autobiography. *Journal of Personality and Social Psychology, 62*(6), 1003–1015. doi:10.1037/0022-3514.62.6.1003

McCall, M. W., Lombardo, M. M., & Morrison, A. M. (1988). *The lessons of experience: How successful executives develop on the job.* Lexington, MA: Lexington Books.

McKenna, R. B., Boyd, T. N., & Yost, P. R. (2007). Learning agility in clergy: Understanding the personal strengths and situational factors that enable pastors to learn from experience. *Journal of Psychology and Theology, 35*(3), 190-201.

McKenna, R. B., Yost, P. R., & Boyd, T. N. (2007). Leadership development and clergy: Understanding the events and lessons that shape pastoral leaders. *Journal of Psychology and Theology, 35*(3), 179–189.

Merriam, S. B. (1998). *Qualitative research and case study applications in education.* San Francisco, CA: Jossey-Bass.

Merriam, S.B. (2002). *Qualitative research in practice: Examples for discussion and analysis.* San Francisco, CA: Jossey-Bass.

Merriam, S. B. (2009). *Qualitative research: A guide to design and implementation.* San Francisco, CA: Jossey-Bass.

Moustakas, C. (1994). *Phenomenological research methods.* Thousand Oaks, CA: SAGE.

Nelson, K. W., Oliver, M., & Capps, F. (2006). Becoming a supervisor: Doctoral student perceptions of the training experience. *Counselor Education & Supervision, 46*(1), 17–31.

Northouse, P. G. (2010). *Leadership: Theory and practice* (5th ed.). Los Angeles, CA: SAGE.

Patton, M. Q. (1990). *Qualitative evaluation and research methods* (2nd ed.). Newbury Park, CA: SAGE.

Patton, M. Q. (2002). Two decades of developments in qualitative inquiry: A personal, experiential perspective. *Qualitative Social Work, 1*(3), 261–283.

Perlman, B., & Hartman, A. (1987). Psychologist administrators in community mental health organizations. *Professional Psychology: Research and Practice, 18*(1), 36–41.

Piaget, J., & Inhelder, B. (1969). *The psychology of the child.* New York, NY: Basic Books.

Quinn, R. E., Spreitzer, G. M., & Brown, M. V. (2000). Changing others through changing ourselves. *Journal of Management Inquiry, 9*(2), 147–164. doi:10.1177/105649260092010

Report of the National Task Force on Mental Health/Mental Retardation Administration. (1979). *Administration in Mental Health, 6*(4), 269–289.

Robinson, G. S., & Wick, C. W. (1992). Executive development that makes a business difference. *Human Resource Planning, 15*(1), 63–76.

Schwandt, T. A. (1994). Constructivist, interpretivist approaches to human inquiry. In N. K. Denzin & Y. S. Lincoln (Eds.), *Handbook of qualitative research* (pp. 118–137). Thousand Oaks, CA: SAGE.

Sergiovanni, T. J. (2007). *Rethinking leadership: A collection of articles.* Thousand Oaks, CA: Corwin Press.

Slater, C. L. (2003). Generativity versus stagnation: An elaboration of Erikson's adult stage of human development. *Journal of Adult Development, 10*(1), 53–65.

Sluyter, G. V. (1995). Mental health leadership training: A survey of state directors. *The Journal of Mental Health Administration, 22*(2), 201–204.

Tosey, P. (2006, May). *Bateson's levels of learning: A framework for transformative learning?* Paper presented at Universities' Forum for Human Resource Development conference, University of Tilburg, Tilburg, The Netherlands. Retrieved from http://www.ufhrd.co.uk/wordpress/wp-content/uploads/2008/06/12-2_tosey.pdf

Turner, J., & Mavin, S. (2008). What can we learn from senior leader narratives? The strutting and fretting of becoming a leader. *Leadership & Organization Development Journal, 29*(4), 376–391.

Van Manen, M. (1990). *Researching the lived experience: Human science for an action sensitive pedagogy.* Ontario, Canada: State University of New York Press.

Walumbwa, F. O., Avolio, B. J., Gardner, W. L., Wernsing, T. S., & Peterson, S. J. (2008). Authentic leadership: Development and validation of a theory-based measure. *Journal of Management, 34*(1), 89–126.

Waters, J. T., Marzano, R. J., & McNulty, B. A. (2003). *Balanced leadership: What 30 years of research tells us about the effect of leadership on student achievement.* Aurora, CO: Mid-continent Research for Education and Learning.

Watkins, C. E. (1990). Development of the psychotherapy supervisor. *Psychotherapy: Theory, Research, Practice, Training, 27*(4), 553–560.

Watzlawick, P., Weakland, J. H., & Fisch, R. (1974). *Change: Principles of problem formation and problem resolution.* New York, NY: Norton.

Webb, P.K. (1980). Teaching methods: Learning applications. *Theory into Practice, 19*(2), 93–97.

APPENDIX A: INTERVIEW QUESTIONS

Category 1: Experiences

(1) Describe the experience of transitioning from a clinician to an executive director.

(2) What has the experience taught you about yourself?

(3) What lessons have you have learned?

(4) Over the course of your tenure as a leader, what aspects of your job or experiences during your job have forced you to learn and grow the most?

(5) What about each of those aspects or experiences of your job made them areas in which you feel you need to grow?

(6) What did these aspects or experiences of your job reveal to you about yourself as a leader?

(7) Describe the change you have experienced as a person through this experience.

Category 2: Developmental Process

(8) Would you describe the experience as cyclical or linear? Explain.

(9) How did these experiences and the learning that took place change the way you lead?

(10) Describe yourself as a leader before you went through the above experience and after you had learned from it.

(11) Describe how you saw yourself when you first began the job and how you see yourself now.

(12) How would you characterize this change (from clinician to director)?

Category 3: Resources

(13) Describe the resources that helped you grow.

(14) Why were each of these resources so important?

After an initial interview with these questions, I conducted a second interview to clarify any information and also to ask the subjects to describe, in their own words, their overall experience of development.

www.ingramcontent.com/pod-product-compliance
Lightning Source LLC
Chambersburg PA
CBHW080819180526
45168CB00006B/2502